Empowerment

T0298534

'Empowerment' is a term in widespread use today and one that is often considered to be a self-evident good. Here, McLaughlin explores its emergence in the 1960s through to its rise in the 1990s and ubiquity in present day discourse and interrogates its social status, paying particular attention to social policy, social work and health and social care discourse. He argues that a focus on empowerment has superseded the notion of political subjects exercising power autonomously.

This innovative volume:

- Discusses the relationship between concepts of empowerment and power, as they have been understood historically.
- Analyses changes in the conception and meaning of empowerment in relation to the shifting social and political landscape.
- Acknowledges the positive impact empowerment strategies have had on those who have campaigned to be empowered and also on those who have seen their role as being to help empower others.
- Highlights ways in which talk about empowerment can actually work in such a way as to further disempower those already marginalised.

Critically examining how 'empowerment' has become embedded in contemporary social and political life, this work offers a discussion of the term's multiple meanings, what it actually entails, and how it constructs and positions those being empowered and those empowering.

Kenneth McLaughlin is Senior Lecturer in the Research Institute for Health and Social Change, Manchester Metropolitan University, UK.

Routledge key themes in health and society

Empowerment
A critique

Kenneth McLaughlin

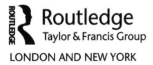

Taylor & Francis Group

LONDON AND NEW YORK

First published 2016
by Routledge
4 Park Square, Milton Park, Abingdon, Oxon OX14 4RN
605 Third Avenue, New York, NY 10017

First issued in paperback 2023

Routledge is an imprint of the Taylor & Francis Group, an informa business

British Library Cataloguing-in-Publication Data
A catalogue record for this book is available from the British Library

Library of Congress Cataloging in Publication Data
McLaughlin, Kenneth, author.
Empowerment : a critique / Kenneth McLaughlin.
  p. ; cm. – (Routledge key themes in health and society)
  Includes bibliographical references and index.
  I. Title. II. Series: Routledge key themes in health and society.
  [DNLM: 1. Health Policy. 2. Truth Disclosure. 3. Power (Psychology)
  4. Public Policy. 5. Social Work. WA 525]
  RA418
  362.1–dc23   2015031877

ISBN: 978-1-03-256972-7 (pbk)
ISBN: 978-1-138-81961-0 (hbk)
ISBN: 978-1-315-74433-9 (ebk)

DOI: 10.4324/9781315744339

Typeset in Times New Roman
by Wearset Ltd, Boldon, Tyne and Wear

Publisher's Note
The publisher has gone to great lengths to ensure the quality of this reprint but
points out that some imperfections in the original copies may be apparent.

Contents

Acknowledgements

I would like to thank those who have read and commented on various chapters of this book as it developed: Josie Appleton, Concetta Banks, Martin King, Ann McLaughlin, Rachel Robbins, Sandy Starr, Gemma Yarwood and Chris Yianni. As ever, I owe a great debt to Ian Parker for his help and advice as the book progressed and for his feedback on an earlier draft.

This book would have been unlikely to have been completed without the time made available to me by Comast. A word of thanks is therefore due to all the children and parents who, like myself, spend a considerable amount of their time at MAC, where most of this book was written, and who have kept me company both mornings and evening as I worked on it – you know who you are.

In the course of writing this book I have reproduced extracts from some of my earlier academic work: McLaughlin, K. (2014) 'Empowering the People: "Empowerment" and the British Journal of Social Work, 1971–99', *Critical and Radical Social Work*, vol. 2, no. 2, pp. 203–216 (by permission of The Policy Press); McLaughlin, K. (2015) 'Advocacy Research and Social Policy: Action for Children and the National Society for the Prevention of Cruelty to Children as Case Studies', *International Journal of Sociology and Social Policy*, vol. 35, issue 3/4, pp. 239–251 (by permission of Emerald Group Publishing). I also owe a thank you to all the team at the online political and current affairs magazine *Spiked* (www.spiked-online.com), where I first articulated many of the thoughts and ideas that influenced the development of this book.

Introduction

Background

'I want to empower people.' This is a common reply when I ask prospective social work students why they want to become a social worker. The choice of terminology is revealing in that it is reflective of changes within both social work and politics in the contemporary period. In using the specific word 'empowerment' prospective students indicate that they have at least prepared for interview by reading some relevant material; the term pervades the social work literature, with books, articles and various organisational statements routinely declaring that they are in the business of 'empowering' people. The value of, and need to, empower people has also become part of the party political process, promoted by New Labour during its years in power and is now also embraced by the UK Prime Minister David Cameron as being a natural part of a Conservative approach to government (Cameron, 2009).

These developments were encapsulated in a 2012 interview in the UK *Guardian* newspaper with Stella Creasy, Labour MP for Walthamstow. Ms Creasy sees her political role as one in which she gives power and authority to individuals and groups within society (Aitkenhead, 2012). The example she gives is of her decision to get eight of her constituents, who needed new cookers, to buy them collectively as this would reduce the price. Now, that may be a wise and commendable thing to do, but is such a micro issue really the role of an MP as opposed to a more organic community group?[1] Reading this interview in the same week that I had spent several days interviewing prospective students got me thinking about why this term was so popular and from where it emerged. A cursory search of the archives of the *British Journal of Social Work*, arguably the United Kingdom's most prestigious social work academic publication, revealed that the term was one rarely mentioned in the journal during the first two decades of its existence (1971–1990). Today, by contrast, the term proliferates within social work discourse. Initially, it was this aspect of the concept that was the intended focus of my investigation.

I soon began to realise that whilst empowerment's use within social work was a very important area to investigate, in many respects this was but one of many areas within which similar strategies emphasising behaviour change for citizens were manifest. For me, this became, if anything, more important to highlight. After all, whilst social work has been correctly criticised for implementing policies and practices aimed at pacifying and controlling the poor, it is a profession that does entail an overt emphasis on changing the behaviour of those with whom it works. Whether that should be on a more individual and personal level or a more collective and political one is often debated, but both sides agree on the focus on encouraging a change in the behaviour of their clients. However, relatively few of us will be subject to unwanted interventions by social workers, but the newer forms of empowerment affect us all.

The more I looked at such behaviour change strategies, the more I began to see that they were no longer confined to the more political organisations, of which statutory social work is an obvious one. On the contrary, empowerment as behaviour change was far more embedded within society than I had suspected, and therefore a wider range of areas than I had first envisaged are incorporated within the book. Indeed, 'empowerment' as a strategy of intervention is now so embedded within social policy and political discourse that my discussion of how it relates to professional social work forms only a small section of the book. In effect, we have a situation whereby Politics (with a capital P) has become social work, concerned with the micromanagement of everyday life (McLaughlin, 2015).

Empowerment

According to the *American Heritage Dictionary of the English Language,* the word 'empower' can be traced back to at least the mid-seventeenth century when it had the legalistic meaning 'to invest with authority, authorize' and that it also developed to mean 'to enable or permit' (quoted in the Free Dictionary, online). However, its more contemporary usage is rooted in the political movements of the 1960s and 1970s, such as the women's and black liberation groups, most notably in the United States of America (USA). More recently it is a term that has also been utilised by neoconservatives – for example, in the development of 'empowerment zones' – which in reality were about the privatisation of public services (Cruikshank, 1999).

When empowerment began to be discussed in the United Kingdom (UK) during the 1970s, this was often in reference to developments in the USA, and even into the 1980s it did not have the common currency that it enjoys today. It is interesting to note that in Lukes' (2005 [1974]) classic discussion of power, which we consider in Chapter 1, the term empowerment does not appear in the index. It became an increasingly popular term with the New Labour government during its time in power, with one government publication, which contains a foreword by the then Prime Minister, Gordon Brown, and an introduction by then Secretary of State for Communities and Local Government, Hazel Blears, mentioning empowerment 36 times (CLG, 2008). It has become embedded within domestic policies such as health promotion, awareness-raising campaigns and been influenced by psychology and behavioural economics (see Chapters 5, 6 and 7 respectively).

By the mid-1990s empowerment had become a buzz-word not only within Western policy circles but was increasingly being applied to international development. The 1997 New Titles and Development Studies sections of just one publisher (Zen Books) contained the following titles:

> Empowerment: Towards Sustainable Development; Knowledge, Empowerment and Social Transformation: Participatory Research in Africa; Monitoring Family Planning and Reproductive Rights: A Manual for Empowerment; Empowerment and Women's Health: Theory, Methods and Practice; Women and Empowerment: Participation and Decision-Making; Gender in Popular Education: Methods for Empowerment; World Communication: Disempowerment and Self-Empowerment.
>
> (Cheater, 1999, p. 1)

Empowerment has gone global.

Structure of the book

As alluded to above, the shape of the book developed in a way that I did not envisage when I first started to look at the issue of empowerment. Initially, I was specifically interested in what, to my mind at least, were the more obvious manifestations of the term; namely, in the general political process and its incorporation within the discourse and practice of social work. It soon became clear that it would not be possible to discuss empowerment without first discussing the concept of power and how such conceptualisations and practices have changed historically. This proved no easy task given the complexity and disputed meaning of the term, and, even having set aside two chapters to this task, it has to be acknowledged that even this merely scratches the surface of the subject of 'power'. Nevertheless, the discussion of power is meant to situate the remainder of the book as it then looks at the way the discourse of power is often today subsumed under that of empowerment, and of how this latter term, despite having radical political roots, has become institutionalised within political, social policy and social work circles.[2]

The structure of the book is such that whilst it is meant to be read as a whole, each chapter can also be read on its own. In order to achieve this I have incorporated elements from different theoretical discussions at various points throughout the book. To avoid repetition I have tried, where possible, to introduce different theorists at different points so that the theoretical discussion will not merely recap earlier points but further develop them. I also utilise case studies to illustrate my argument, specifically in Chapter 6, but also at other points in the book.

Chapter 1 discusses power as it was conceptualised in the modern age, looking at sovereign power and the work of Niccolo Machiavelli (1469–1527) and Thomas Hobbes (1588–1679). It is reasonable to guess that even those readers engaging with the subject of power for the first time have heard of Machiavelli, his name being synonymous with political duplicity and amoral activity to achieve desired ends. Hobbes may not be so readily known to the new reader but, as we shall see, he has proven highly influential in both the theoretical and practical application of the working of power. Later sociological conceptions of power are also discussed, such as Weber's concept of legitimate power, Parsons' idea of functional power and Lukes' notion of dimensions of power. Power and its relationship to the State and ideology is also discussed with the focus on Marxist-inspired conceptualisations, particularly the work of Althusser and Gramsci. In addition, the idea of 'false consciousness' is discussed, a term that whilst often attributed to those of a Marxist persuasion was not a term used by Marx himself.

The latter writers discussed in Chapter 1 also provide the basis for Chapter 2 where I look at the move away from sovereignty towards that of governmentality. The main focus is on the work of the French thinker Michel Foucault (1926–1984), due not only to the insights his work has given us, many problems with his thinking notwithstanding, but also because of the influence he has had on many within radical social movements, intellectuals and academic circles. As we will see, his analysis of power contained within it a critique of those such as Althusser who held to a more structural analysis of power. His concern with the need to analyse the more micro workings of power resonated with many within the feminist, anti-racist and radical mental health movements as they began to focus on the way in which the 'personal is political'. For similar reasons his work has also been highly influential in the world of social work. Foucault's work, in alerting us to the disciplinary processes that can result from seemingly benign or progressive policies, such as those concerned with psychiatry, is also useful later in the book as we interrogate some of the more contemporary manifestations of empowerment.

In Chapter 3 the focus moves to looking at the change in terminology whereby we begin to see the term empowerment emerge as an adjunct to that of power. The radical roots of the term are highlighted by a specific look at the way it was used within the black, feminist and deaf movements in order to question prevailing social norms and develop new forms of consciousness. I then look at a very contemporary notion, that of 'intersectionality', which was/is an attempt to highlight the way looking at social difference through the prism of one identity – for example, woman or black – can ignore or downplay the different experiences of a white woman to that of a black woman, the former oppressed on account of her gender, the latter on account of both sexism and racism and the way in which they intersect. The tensions and dilemmas within intersectional politics, both theoretically and politically, are discussed in relation to how they have evolved within a changing social and political landscape.

The focus in Chapter 4 remains on the rise of empowerment as a concept and practice but this is done by focusing on its rise and establishment within professional social work discourse. Following a general discussion from the proponents and critics of the term I then concentrate on a specific publication, the *British Journal of Social Work*. This is an important development as not only does it highlight the way in which empowerment became firmly established within social work and social policy discourse, it also alerts us to the way strategies of empowerment can actually entrap people within systems of social control. This is important as it helps situate the remaining half of the book where I detail the expansion of the discourse and practice of empowerment into various areas of social policy. In other words, from its radical roots we begin to see its incorporation and institutionalisation within systems of state governance.

Chapter 5 revisits the concepts of ideology and consciousness-raising discussed in earlier chapters but does so to show the change in discourse from 'consciousness-raising' to 'awareness-raising'. As I will show, this is not a mere semantic change but illustrates both wider social and political developments and how the human subject is viewed today. There is a more individualised and therapeutic notion of the self within the discourse and practice of raising and demonstrating awareness. In addition, a clear moral line is drawn between those who are 'aware' and those considered 'unaware'. Often, awareness-raising campaigns are organised by campaign and charity groups who publish reports with the aim of publicising their specific cause in order to increase their public and political profile and raise further funds to continue their work which ultimately aims to *empower* the specific group for whom they are campaigning (for example, children, older people, victims of domestic violence, etc.).

Whilst often presented and understood as progressive at best, benign at worst, there are many problems with such campaigns, the research they publish and their impact on social policy. Such 'advocacy research' is the subject of Chapter 6, where I use case studies involving two campaigning children's charities, *Action for Children* and the *National Society for the Prevention of Cruelty to Children* respectively, to highlight both the tactics used and negative repercussions that such attempts at raising awareness can have. It is argued that far from being empowering they can, paradoxically, undermine the welfare of the very people they endeavour to help.

Chapter 7 continues the theme of highlighting the way in which empowerment has changed from a more political, collective concept to a more personal and individual one by looking at how its meaning and practice has changed in relation to public health campaigns. By charting the growth of public health concerns and related campaigns to highlight health inequalities, which were initially often resisted by government, through to their incorporation into political discourse and strategy, the changing political and social landscape is once again highlighted. In the process, 'public' health became transformed into a moralistic and individualised 'private' matter in that the weaknesses of the individual became seen as the cause and object of change within health policy.

From a focus on the awareness-raising and health promotion agendas of the previous two chapters, Chapter 8 considers a more recent development within the behaviour change agenda that has become commonly known as the 'politics of Nudge'. Where this differs most from the preceding strategies is in its subterfuge, with insights from behavioural economics and psychology used to develop ways in which to 'nudge' citizens to behave in ways that are better for their well-being, such as contributing to a pension, eating healthier food, stopping smoking and drinking alcohol in moderation. It is often referred to as form of 'libertarian paternalism' – we are merely nudged to make a certain choice, not forced to. The difference between this and the awareness-raising and health promotion tactics of the past is in the way that the 'nudgers' manipulate or organise the environment in such a way that we make the correct choices, as they see it, without us necessarily being aware of it. In other words it is *empowerment by subterfuge*, working on the assumption that we are cognitively impaired citizens.

The conclusion draws all the strands of my argument together, highlighting both the positive and negative outcomes that strategies of empowerment entail. There is a need to be aware of the ideological assumptions and practical consequences surrounding the discourse of empowerment, and to be alert to both the overt and covert workings of power. In other words we need to view empowerment not as a fixed, a priori good, but as embedded within social and political relationships, and therefore as a concept that can be used for either progressive or regressive social policies and social work practices.

As I delved more into the subject of power and empowerment I have to confess to becoming more interested in certain aspects of the debate, and certain writers, than others. This will obviously mean that I have neglected many writers whose work could have added to my discussion. However, it is never possible to include everyone and everything, and I also have to admit that my research was guided more by a concern to educate myself than to write a book for public consumption. However, in so doing I remained aware of the overall aim of my initial interest and project, and felt that so long as I did not veer off at too much of a tangent I could educate both myself and, to at least some extent, the reader. I have certainly achieved the former, although it is obviously for you, as the reader, to judge the latter claim.

Notes

1 Ms Creasy's other main concern is with health inequalities related to lifestyle. I wonder what the empowering MP's thoughts and actions would have been if her constituents had used the money she saved them to buy cheap alcohol or cigarettes. As we will see, a key contemporary manifestation of 'empowerment' centres on encouraging people to adopt 'appropriate' and 'healthy' lifestyles. No doubt that whilst the power she gave them would be seen as good, their exercise of personal power and autonomy would be frowned upon.
2 I use social work not only to refer to statutory or professionally qualified social workers but in the broader sense of those organisations doing forms of 'social' work.

1   Power in modernity

Introduction

If the concept of empowerment is concerned with the distribution of power, it is necessary to detail what is meant when we talk about power. Indeed, 'power' is a word that is so ingrained in political and public discourse that its complexity can often be overlooked. Public discussion is often framed around a polarisation between the powerful and the powerless. It can take a variety of forms; we talk about, *inter alia*, political power, physical power, organisational power, media power and religious power. Sales campaigns often target children in recognition of their 'pester power', which it is hoped will eventually persuade their parents to purchase the desired object for the sake of peace and quiet. In addition, our interactions with our fellow humans are said to be shaped by racialized and gendered power relations whether at the macro, meso or micro level of social interaction. We frequently feel powerless in the face of seemingly insurmountable power, whether from the vagaries of our employer, the financial market, local authorities or other bureaucratic organisations. People can feel powerless to escape abusive relationships and/or economic deprivation. Those fleeing persecution, or merely looking for a better standard of living than is available in their country of birth, will soon feel the power of border control agencies standing in the way of a safe haven and/or economic opportunity.

However, despite its ubiquity, power is a difficult concept to define. In this chapter I explore some of the classical sociological discussions of power, in the process highlighting the complexities, theoretical explanations and material manifestations of power. This is important not only in and of itself but also to situate the later discussion of empowerment and how both terms are interrelated.

Sovereign power

From the power and authority of the Gods (within pantheism), or God (within monotheism), or of major religions such as Christianity and Islam and the earthly religious leaders who were trusted to interpret the 'true message', concerns with power and authority are as old as mankind itself. It is beyond the scope of this book to cover such a history, and for our purposes the focus will be on more modern conceptions of power. Even here it is not possible to draw a clear line, a total break with the past when a new theory emerged unencumbered from the thoughts of the past. Nevertheless, we have to start somewhere, and a good place to do so is with the thought of the sixteenth-century Florentine, Niccolo Machiavelli, and the seventeenth-century Englishman, Thomas Hobbes. This is due to Hobbes being regarded by many as articulating the form of modern secular government, with his emphasis on a central, sovereign authority that replaced the previous religious and feudal systems of rule. Machiavelli is often drawn upon, sometimes unwittingly, by those who consider that we are now in a postmodern age in which power is said to be dispersed throughout the social body, and which therefore entails the need for an analysis of systems, or strategies, of power.

In the centuries following their work, it was arguably the thought of Hobbes that had the most impact on future thinkers, with his premises being utilised in many modern conceptualisations of power. Nevertheless, in the twentieth century the influence of Machiavelli has arguably taken more hold on the popular and public imagination. Many who will never have read any of Machiavelli's work will be aware that his name is synonymous with political machinations, betrayal and strategic manoeuvring. Indeed, Peter Mandelson, who played a key role within the UK Labour Party during the 1980s and 1990s, including a time as its 'director of communications' or 'media adviser', was often portrayed as a Machiavellian figure, the 'spin doctor' manipulating both the media and politicians in such a way as to achieve the goals of government.

In addition to having resonance within public discourse, Machiavelli's work has received increased attention within social and political theoretical analyses, particularly from the 1950s onwards, proving popular with those of a more postmodern persuasion who draw on the way that his analysis of power focused on strategies of power, being concerned with the complex interactions within relations of power, as opposed to the more causal and linear mechanisms of power found in the work of many from Hobbes onwards. We will look at this in more detail in Chapter 2 when we discuss the work and influence of Michel Foucault. For now, it is necessary to give a brief account of the thinking of both Hobbes and Machiavelli.

Hobbes developed his thinking in a period that had witnessed great social turmoil. Seventeenth-century England had experienced a Civil War and Hobbes was greatly concerned with the need for a return to social order, something that he saw as best achieved by the unification of power in a single sovereign authority. For Hobbes the choice was stark. We could have a modern world where civility, sovereignty and rule flourished or we could have one in which,

> there is no place for industry; because the fruit thereof is uncertain: and consequently no culture of the earth; no navigation, not use of the commodities that may be imposed by the sea; no commodious building; no instruments of moving, and removing, such things as require much force; no knowledge of the face of the earth; no account of time; no arts; no letters; no society; and

which is worst of all, continual fear and danger of violent death; and the life of man, solitary, poor, nasty, brutish, and short.

(Hobbes, 2008 [1651]), p. 84)

Hobbes was of the view that a lack of sovereign authority would lead to the breakdown of civil society and reduce us to the state of nature, the pitting of 'all against all'. However, there is no anthropological referent for such a negation. For some, Hobbes' conception is seen as fulfilling the role of myth, a theorisation of the possible dystopian society. As such he has been criticised for offering an oversimplified representation concerned not only with the 'state of nature' but also the 'state of order', in which 'each was equally fanciful but both served a strategic purpose: that of producing legitimation for a political community' (Clegg, 1989, p. 26).

This more pragmatic reason for the centralisation of power was bolstered by Hobbes' view of humanity's ability for moral reasoning. Hobbes had faith in scientific claims to rational intelligence. He firmly believed that 'armed with the right method, and further armed with opportunity, man could construct a political order as timeless as a Euclidian theorem' (Wolin, 1960, p. 243).

Society, for Hobbes, comes into existence when individuals contract out of the state of nature and give up some of their freedoms for security and peace. His conceptualisation differs from Rousseau's 'social contract' in that the former focuses on the restraint of natural impulses by the sovereign whereas the latter has more of an emphasis on the creation of common social rules (Rousseau, 1998 [1762]). The renunciation of violent means to pursue one's goals and desires is replaced by the establishment of a set of rules, customs and laws to which all must abide. The place where such power should reside in order to ensure such compliance is, in Hobbes' view, the body of the sovereign, in a secular rather than a religious authority. Such a situation relies on a notion of political community, of a body of people with a common interest in, and identification with, the social and political organisation of the day. Without the people there can be no sovereign. In other words, Hobbes was aware that a modicum of consent was necessary for a stable government and society. This is illustrated on the front cover of the 1651 edition of Hobbes' most famous work, *Leviathan*, which represents the sovereign as a large figure overlooking an orderly, but by contrast, miniscule, civil society. However, there is another feature of the frontispiece worth noting. As Wolin (1960) points out,

The sovereign's powerful body is, so to speak, not his own; its outline is completely filled in by the miniature figures of his subjects. He exists, in other words, only through them. Equally important, each subject is clearly discernible in the body of the sovereign. The citizens are not swallowed up in an anonymous mass, nor sacramentally merged into a mystical body. Each remains a discrete individual and each retains his identity in an absolute way.

(p. 266)

In essence, what the image represents is the identity of the subject as an individual but an individual whose identity is subsumed within the body of the sovereign. The sovereign is the people in another state, but 'not in a mystical way but as the result of a symbolic translation of voice: the social contract' (Clegg, 1960, p. 27).

The political community envisaged by Hobbes is seen as being like an extension outwards from family, to locality, to the political community of citizens, something that was integral to the establishment of the nation-state and political citizens. Power is concentrated in 'one man or upon one assembly of men, that may reduce all their wills, by plurality of voices, unto one will' (Hobbes, 2008 [1651]), p. 114). This 'one will' representing the plurality of voices is the sovereign/state power: Leviathan. The sovereign/state is the parent to the family, maintaining order and disciplining when necessary. Hobbes articulated a theory of power whereby its centralisation in sovereign or state power could achieve social stability and order. This new combination of state power and resources, coupled with a discursive framework within which it was situated represented 'modernity' (Bauman, 1982).

As mentioned above, Hobbes was concerned with the need for social stability to prevent the outbreak of civil disorder and war and this influenced his articulation of the need for absolute power, akin to a dictatorship, situated with the sovereign. In the time since Hobbes wrote, democracies have attempted to place restrictions on the use of arbitrary state power against its citizens. However, at times of crisis it is not uncommon to hear calls for such rights of citizenship to be revoked in the name of peace or social order. At such times it is Hobbes' Leviathan that is being invoked.

Machiavelli and 'strategies of power'

Power, for Machiavelli, was not conceived in the instrumental way of Hobbes, as the power of a man to obtain some future good, but in terms of expediency and strategy. Rather than legislating for a social contract, Machiavelli would analyse and interpret a strategy. Where Hobbes conceived of power in terms of motion, causality, agency and action, Machiavelli was more concerned with revealing the workings of power, of discovering the rules of the game. In *The Prince*, Machiavelli (2009 [1532]) provides a detailed ethnography of power in terms of strategic effectiveness with little regard for the morality of any such strategy. The strategies

> are neither good or bad, their only purpose is their effectiveness. They flow from no principle of sovereignty; they serve no principle of sovereignty; they reproduce no principle of sovereignty. Machiavelli does not serve power: he merely describes its strategies as he sees it at work within the arena of the palace. Power does not belong to anyone nor to any place; it is not something that princes necessarily have; it is no Leviathan. Power is simply the effectiveness for achieving for oneself a greater scope for action

than for others implicated by one's strategies. Power is not any thing nor is it necessarily inherent in any one; it is a tenuously produced and reproduced effect which is contingent upon the strategic competencies and skills of actors who would be powerful.

(Clegg, 1989, pp. 32–33)

The Prince embodied a change in the intended audience for political treatises. With the decline of republican institutions in mid-fifteenth century Italy and the rise of the rule of princes, political publications tended to be addressed directly to the princes rather than to the whole body of citizens. As a consequence, the individual citizen is ignored and all attention concentrated on that of the prince. In *The Foundations of Modern Political Thought*, his remarkably detailed two-volume history of both the renaissance and the reformation, Skinner (1978a, 1978b) notes how *The Prince* can be read as an extended job application. After the overthrow of the Florentine Republic and the return to power of the Medici, Machiavelli had lost his job as a public servant. With *The Prince* he hoped to find favour with the Medici and regain political employment.

Nevertheless, Machiavelli was at times hostile to the idea of monarchical government. In the *Discourses* he states his belief that whilst 'there are and have been any number of princes, but of good and wise ones there have been but few' (quoted in Skinner, 1978a, p. 159), and also that government by the people is better than government by princes as the populace makes fewer mistakes than do princes and therefore can be more trusted.

Despite the apparent differences in the *Discourses* and *The Prince*, both are concerned with advising on and shaping political opinion, the former being addressed to the whole body of citizens, the latter to individual princes. His support for 'reprehensible' actions is on the basis that they 'are often unavoidable if the freedom of the commonwealth is to be preserved – a value which is thus allowed to override any rival considerations in favour of clemency, justice or the other conventional virtues of political life' (Skinner, 1978a, p. 184). As a consequence it is unsurprising that Machiavelli is often read as believing that 'the end justifies the means', although the verbs he uses are 'accusare and scusare. The action itself accuses, but its outcome excuses (rather than justifies) its performance' (ibid., emphasis in original).

Many of Machiavelli's insights are pertinent to contemporary political strategy. In *The Prince* he warns that 'one may be very strong in armed forces, yet in entering a province one has always need of the goodwill of the natives' (2009 [1532], p. 5). This necessity, which in contemporary discourse is termed 'the winning of hearts and minds', is something that was palpably not achieved by the USA-led military invasions of Afghanistan and Iraq during the first decade of the twenty-first century.

This need for the goodwill of the natives did not mean that Machiavelli was averse to the exercise of harsh and brutal punishment by the Prince, even if it meant incurring a reputation as a cruel master. Indeed, for him, the reproach of cruelty should not unduly bother the Prince, and as long as the examples of such cruelty were relatively few the prince 'will be more merciful than those who, through too much mercy, allow disorders to arise, from which follow murders or robberies; for these are wont to injure the whole people, whilst those executions which originate with a prince offend the individual only' (ibid., p. 59). Whilst he agrees that it is better to be both loved and feared, he notes that such a balance is difficult to achieve and therefore if the choice is between one or the other 'it is much safer to be feared than loved' (ibid., p. 60). To be most successful an 'economy of violence' is necessary whereby strategies of power need to know not only when to resort to violence but also when to withdraw.

Weber and legitimate power

Max Weber was arguably one of the most influential sociologists of the twentieth century, his work on power being especially pertinent to the development of our understanding of the concept. Weber made the important distinction between power as authority and power as coercion. There were two aspects of authority that he considered central to historical types of domination: first, was the ruler's authority viewed as legitimate by those subject to it, and second, did such authority rely on the rise of an administrative apparatus containing personnel who will see that the ruler's commands are carried out. This administrative system mediates between the rulers and the people. In modern Western democracies the legal system, police and local authorities, amongst others, can be seen as ensuring that the commands of those in authority are carried out.

Within modern societies Weber saw domination as comprising elements of each of three historical forms of legitimate domination: charismatic domination, traditional domination and rational-legal domination. Traditional domination refers to the 'age old rules and powers' that are held to give the ruler, such as the monarch and aristocracy in feudal societies, their authority and concomitant power. Deference to authority in traditional societies is not due to an enacted legal system but rather from the ruler's position and the authority deemed to be inherent within that position. In contrast, it is precisely adherence to the legality of enacted rules that characterises 'legal-domination'. Modern Western democracies can be viewed as examples of legal-domination whereby compliance with the commands of authority figures is expected on the grounds that their power has been legitimated on principles of law, and unlike sovereign power even those holding power are subject to the same legal constraints as those to whom they issue commands. Charismatic domination refers to 'a certain quality of an individual's personality which is considered extraordinary and treated as capable of having supernatural, superhuman, or exceptional powers and qualities' (Weber, 1978 [1922], p. 241). Weber had in mind leaders whose right to rule could be based on either divine origin, such as religious leaders, or conversely, those who emerge from the existing population but command obedience due to the populace seeing them as possessing heroic or mystical powers. Morrison (2006) gives Mahatma Gandhi's struggle to end British colonial rule in India as an explicit example of charismatic leadership. Gandhi, despite lacking political power and combat resources still managed to mobilise a large resistance movement. His behaviour and charismatic personality allowed him to claim to represent a higher ethical order than that of the British colonial rulers.

Weber considered authority to be the legitimate use of power, for example, when the police use their power to arrest a suspect and most citizens view that as a legitimate use of state power, then this is an aspect of authority. Power as coercion, on the other hand, involves force, often with the threat of violence, in order to make someone act the way the other person wants them to. The principle of legitimacy then was crucial for Weber; how legitimate was the ruler's power and, more importantly, how did those subject to such power perceive it to be a legitimate form of power. Whilst not a pre-given – there are many examples of serious social unrest against state power – the use of power by those in authority is often accepted as legitimate by the majority of the population. As mentioned above, the powers of arrest and detention given to the police and judiciary are, for the most part, accepted within Western democracies. However, at times, the acceptance of authority can seem equivocal. For example, social work is arguably one of the most controversial professions in the UK, often being castigated for failing to protect children and vulnerable adults from serious harm, and conversely for at times intervening too readily into the private sphere of family life. Nevertheless, despite such public opprobrium, it is generally accepted that there is a legitimate role for social workers in using their statutory powers to intervene into people's lives, subject to certain criteria being met, irrespective of the wishes of those subject to the intervention; their authority to intervene in family life, whilst subject to some constraint and unease, is accepted by the majority of the population. The debate is over the specifics of when such intervention is justified, not over the right for social workers, as proxies of the state, to hold such power. Similarly, when a schoolteacher tells a child what to do or a manager instructs an employee to carry out certain tasks it is generally accepted that to do so is a legitimate use of power as authority.

When such authority is unquestioned social stability is relatively easy to maintain. However, when it is not accepted as legitimate social disorder can arise; the political conflict in the North of Ireland from the late 1960s to the mid-1990s can be seen as arising due to a sizeable proportion of the population of the six counties refusing to accept the legitimacy of the authority of the British state.

It is important to note here that Weber's main concern is with political power and how it operated in different historical epochs. In this respect, although he implicitly acknowledges the internalisation of power by virtue of the acceptance of authority as legitimate, his analysis can be seen as a broad sociological, top-down approach to power culminating in its manifestation in modernity. He was influenced by Marx's work on the primacy of class relations. From a traditional Marxist viewpoint the concern is not with authority per se, than with authority as it manifests itself within a given society's relations of production. For Marx, in a society with a capitalist mode of production, authority is a relationship of dependence for the worker.

Weber was concerned to develop a theory that saw class relations as far more stratified and complex than Marx's 'proletariat vs bourgeoisie' dualism. Weber highlighted three dimensions of power that affected an individual's life chances; economic power, communal power and authoritarian power. Economic power was a result of 'class situation', i.e. where the individual is located within capitalist market relations, communal power was linked to social status which came from the amount of prestige an individual holds within his or her society, something that is heavily influenced by that society's prevailing norms, for example prestige based on ethnicity, gender, occupation, title etc. So, in modern capitalist economies, manual labour is given less prestige than skilled, professional work such as the legal or medical professions. His work on social stratification sought to identify the way such different power relations operated within society in such a way that they shaped both the individual and the social structure. In looking at authoritarian power, Weber was interested in the way in which authority, closely linked to bureaucratic power, was distributed within society. Within the workplace, and indeed wider society, there are those who issue commands and those who are expected to obey such instruction. Taken together, the economic, communal and authority aspects of power to a great extent shape the life chances of individuals within modern societies.

Parsons and functional power

For Parsons (1957), power is functional for society as a whole but it is dependent on the institutionalisation of authority. Whilst acknowledging the difficulty in obtaining definitional or conceptual clarity, he did, however, believe that at its core it was about the ability of individuals or collectives to achieve their desired goals, especially when such goals were obstructed by the resistance of opposing forces. However, Parsons did not see power as something to be fought out between competing actors or groups in some zero-sum game, whereby there was a fixed quantity of power in existence and the gaining of power by one must therefore entail a loss of power by another. He saw power as something that facilitated the performance of function for the behalf of society as a system.

Parson sees power as analogous to money in the economy, it is 'the *means* of acquiring control of the factors in effectiveness; it is not itself one of these factors, any more than in the economic case money is a factor of production' (1963, p. 234, emphasis in original). It is, like money, 'a circulating medium, moving back and forth over the boundaries of the polity' (p. 245). Power then,

> is generalized capacity to secure the performance of binding obligations by units in a system of collective organization when the obligations are legitimized with reference to their bearing on collective goals and where in case of recalcitrance there is a presumption of enforcement by negative situational sanctions – whatever the actual agency of that enforcement.
>
> (Parsons, 1963, p. 237)

To be effective, power is also required to be symbolically reinforced and legitimised in order that obligations are binding and can be enforced if necessary.

Authority, for Parsons, is the right to assert priority of decision over others. This can be situational, for example the power of the social worker over certain of their clients does not extend outside the working day. Authority, then, 'is essentially the institutional code within which the use of power as medium is organized and legitimized' (Parsons, 1963, p. 243). Parsons, in effect, idealised society as being akin to a well-oiled machine where everyone has a vested interest in keeping oiled.

These early sociological perspectives on power set the scene for subsequent writers who developed varying dimensions of power.

Dimensions of power

In developing a three dimensional view of power, Lukes (2005) not only highlighted the weaknesses of the prevailing 'pluralist' view of power, which for him was too one-dimensional in scope, he also felt that many criticisms of the pluralist approach, whilst yielding some insights, nevertheless were themselves limited in scope, being merely two-dimensional. The pluralist approach tended to emphasise behaviour, the process of decision making and observable (overt) conflict. According to Lukes (2005), this is a 'one-dimensional view of power as it involves a focus on *behaviour* in the making of *decisions* on *issues* over which there is an observable *conflict* of subjective *interests*, seen as express policy preferences, revealed by political participation (p. 19, emphasis in original).

The main criticism of this model is that it does not take into account the role of *non-decision making* in the exercise of power, for example in the way that certain issues can be sidelined or ignored. For example, Bacharah and Baratz see the emphasis on behaviour as failing to take into account 'the fact that power may be, and often is, exercised by confining the scope of decision-making to relatively "safe" issues' (quoted in Lukes, 2005, p. 22). In this respect, any satisfactory account of the workings of power must involve an examination of both decision making and non-decision making, decision-making being 'a choice among alternative modes of action' whereas a non-decision involves 'a decision that results in the suppression or thwarting of a latent or manifest challenge to the values or interests of the decision-maker' (ibid.).

Whilst seeing such a two-dimensional approach as being an improvement on the previous one-sided viewpoint, Lukes (2005) points out that the two-dimensional approach shares with the pluralist approach a focus on overt or covert *observable* conflict, something that he views as inadequate on three counts. First, its critique of behaviourism is too limited; it still studies *actual behaviour* and *concrete decisions*. It attempts to,

> assimilate all cases of exclusion of potential issues from the political agenda to the paradigm of a decision. Decisions are choices consciously and intentionally made by individuals between alternatives, whereas the bias of the system can be mobilized, recreated and reinforced in ways that are neither consciously chosen nor the intended result of particular individuals' choices.
>
> (p. 25)

Second, the focus on observable conflict inadequately considers processes of manipulation and authority. There is a failure to acknowledge the way the powerful can influence, shape and determine the wants, desires and values of the powerless. In this respect, alongside the one-sided pluralist view, the two-dimensional view of power conceptualises it as necessitating actual conflict. This is a mistake because, as Lukes argues, it 'is to ignore the crucial point that the most effective and insidious use of power is to prevent such conflict from arising in the first place' (ibid., p. 27).

Third, and linked to the second, is the insistence that non-decision making power can only exist when there are genuine grievances that are prevented from entry into the political process. This not only raises the question of just what exactly constitutes a grievance and who decides, it also assumes that 'if people feel no grievances, then they have no interests that are harmed by the use of power' (ibid., p. 28). This misses the important point that people's perceptions, values and preferences can be influenced and shaped by prevailing power interests and institutions. As Lukes puts it, 'To assume that the absence of grievance equals genuine consensus is simply to rule out the possibility of false or manipulated consensus by definitional fiat' (ibid.).

Here, Lukes is bringing in concepts such as hegemony, ideology and false consciousness. A focus on intentional and effective acts of power can miss the hidden operations of power, something that, as we will discuss in the following chapter, writers such as Foucault and Bourdieu were to detail in great depth. Clegg (1989) argues that this point is actually well illustrated by Wrong (1979) even as he tries to claim the opposite. Wrong argues:

> I do not see how we can avoid restricting the term power to intentional and effective acts of influence by some persons on other persons. It may be readily acknowledged that intentional effects to influence others often produce unintended as well as intended effects on their behaviour – a dominating and over-protective mother does not intend to feminize the character of her son. But all social interaction produces such unintended effects – a boss does not mean to plunge an employee into despair by greeting him somewhat distractedly in the morning, nor does a woman mean to arouse a man's sexual interest by paying polite attention to his conversation at a cocktail party.
>
> (p. 4)

Clegg suggests Wrong could hardly have chosen worse examples to make his case as each illustrates the opposite of his argument: the hidden workings of structural and ideological power such as class relations in the employer/employee scenario, femininity and masculinity discourses in the mother/son scenario and sexual politics in the cocktail party interaction. Wrong fails to acknowledge the pre-existing power dynamics that are in place and which actors can take into consideration in deciding how, if at all, to act.

Whilst it is easy to see where Clegg is coming from, his position also illustrates the problem with the blurring of boundaries and destabilising of binaries inherent within much postmodern/poststructural thought and political activism which we discuss in subsequent chapters. All informal interactions can be seen as political to such an extent that politics can lose any sense of meaning. After all, if everything is political then nothing is, or nothing is any more political than anything else. In addition, sexual attraction/flirting gets removed from being part of social life to an arena for political sanction, as can be seen in the plethora of 'codes of conduct' within universities and workplaces most notably in the UK and USA (Hume, 2015). In Chapter 6 we will see how the blurring of boundaries in the case of what constitutes child maltreatment can prove problematic both for social policy and those children who are indeed being abused to a level that warrants external intervention in order to protect them.

In acknowledging that there is no all-embracing concept of power Clegg (1989) nevertheless argues that it is possible to group them into three family groupings of 'dispositional, agency, and facilitative concepts of power' (p. xv) which he attempts to order within a concept of circuits of power. The influence of Lukes on Clegg's notions of power is clear. Indeed Clegg's main concern is to develop a theoretical understanding of power, which, whilst indebted to Lukes, seeks to provide a text that also incorporated more recent debates that have arisen from critiques from influential academic disciplines such as postmodernism and poststructuralism.

Power, ideology and the state

In his paper, *Ideology and Ideological State Apparatuses,* Louis Althusser highlighted the way state institutions such as the school, church and army teach knowledge, but knowledge of a specific kind, that which ensures '*subjection to the ruling ideology* or the mastery of its "practice"' (2001, p. 89, emphasis in original). This subjection is necessary in order for the reproduction of the beliefs and skills necessary for the continuation of the capitalist system:

> the State (and its existence in its apparatus) has no meaning except as a function of *State power*. The whole of the political class struggle revolves around the State. By which I mean around the possession, i.e. the seizure and conservation of State power by a certain class or an alliance between class or class fractions.
>
> (Ibid., p. 94, emphasis in original)

In conceptualising the state as repressive Althusser is following in the Marxist tradition of Lenin, Marx and Engels. In *The State and Revolution*, Lenin (1994 [1917]) saw the state as the creation of the ruling class with its *raison d'être* being to execute the will of its creators. In *The Communist Manifesto,* Marx and Engels (1996 [1872]) describe the state as being the executive committee of the bourgeoisie. However, elsewhere, in *The Housing Question,* Engels writes that 'the state is still to a certain extent a power hovering over society, which for that very reason represents the collective interests of society and not those of a single class' (quoted in Steinmetz, 1993, p. 82). Whilst in *The Origin of the Family, Private Property and the State,* he also states that 'periods occur in which warring classes balance each other so nearly that the state power, an ostensible mediator, acquires for the moment a certain degree of independence from both' (Engels, 2004 [1884], p. 159).

From this it is clear that they do not view the state as being merely a repressive entity. Scholars of Marxism have debated the nuances, apparent inconsistencies and implications of such works for some time and in much detail. This is something Nigan (1996) considers, and he summarises Engels' view as giving us the notion of the state as an entity that 'performs repressive functions but [which] was brought into being in order to [also] protect common interests and perform social functions' (p. 13). This seems to stand in contrast to Lenin's view that the state is a creation of the ruling class. For Engels there was not one creative moment in the repressive state but two, and these were quite distinct: '*the genesis of the political power* and its *appropriation by the economically dominant class*' (Nigan, 1996, p. 13, emphasis in original). Nigan goes on to summarise the apparent contradictions by pointing out that in the above statements the claim being made is a simple one in that it is was when economic production relations reached a certain point of historical development that the conditions for the emergence of political power were created. Once such power had arisen it was simultaneously appropriated by the dominant class.

From this we could argue that the centralised state, Leviathan, did not *arise* as an instrument of class oppression but that as economic power and political power became entwined it developed into an apparatus to favour the bourgeoisie over the proletariat.

Althusser developed Marx's theory of the State, explicitly arguing that there is a need to differentiate between State power and State apparatus. Here he clearly owes a debt to Gramsci (1971) who had previously used the term 'Repressive State Apparatus' under which he included not only the Church and schools but also the trade unions. Althusser (2001) differentiated between the Repressive State Apparatus (RSA) (which includes the government, army, police, courts, prisons etc.) and what he termed Ideological State Apparatuses (ISA) under which he included,

> the religious ISA (the system of the different Churches), the educational ISA (the system of the different public and private 'Schools'), the family ISA, the legal ISA, the political ISA (the political system, including the different Parties), the trade union ISA, the communications ISA (press, radio and television, etc.), the cultural ISA (Literature, the Arts, sports, etc.).
>
> (2001, p. 96)

The difference between the Repressive State Apparatus and the Ideological State Apparatus is that whilst there is one RSA, there is a plurality of ISAs. Whilst there is some debate as to whether they belong in the public or private domains, straddle both, or indeed whether the RSA transcends the public/private distinction, the crucial difference between them is how they function. For Althusser, 'the Repressive State Apparatus functions "by violence", whereas the Ideological State Apparatuses *function "by ideology"*' (p. 97, emphasis in original).

In the pre-capitalist historical period the Church performed the role of transmitting the favoured ideas and values of the day, but as capitalism developed and society became less cohesive more organisations performed this role – for example the school, family, media etc. – although for Althusser the educational system had replaced the Church as the dominant ideological apparatus. The School

> takes children from every class at infant-school age, and then for years and years in which the child is most 'vulnerable', squeezed between the family State apparatus and the educational State apparatus, it drums into them, whether it uses new or old methods, a certain amount of 'know-how' wrapped in ruling ideology.
>
> (p. 104)

The school, for Althusser, is now coupled with the family in the same way that the Church was coupled with the family in the past. The use of the educational system to pursue political ends can be seen today, with it being used to promote government sponsored forms of health and behaviour, for example around 'healthy eating', 'anti-bullying' and 'anti-discriminatory' polices and guidance, which are, at best, still examples of state sponsored ideology being transmitted to children via the education system, at worst a new form of state regulation of admissible thoughts and behaviours

Power, hegemony and false consciousness

Whilst Marx concentrated his analysis on the economic base within the capitalist social structure, many of his followers also began an analysis of the superstructure, offering critical analyses of the economy's relations with culture, class and power. Perhaps the most influential of these was the Italian Marxist Antonio Gramsci (1891–1937). A concern for many Marxist writers since the October 1917 revolution has been to try and explain the failure of the working class in other advanced capitalist countries to fulfil its historical role and instigate communist revolution. Gramsci's concept of hegemony was one of the first, and arguably one of the most influential, theoretical attempts to provide such an explanation.

Hegemony has been defined as 'a synthesis of political, intellectual and moral leadership in which a class passes from defending its own "corporate" interests to unifying and directing all other social groups' (Swingewood, 2000, p. 118). It is generally understood to involve the successful enlistment and reproduction of the active consent of oppressed or dominated groups. For Gramsci, the working class did not passively absorb an overpowering bourgeois social structure; on the contrary they actively acquiesced to the reproduction of bourgeois society. This does not discount the role of dissent, both consent and coercion are elements within a hegemonic social order, however, whilst force plays a part in maintaining the status quo it is not the dominant means of enforcing it.

For Swingewood, Gramsci's

> concept of hegemony is analytically valuable for its rejection of the positivistic conception of the economic as the 'basis' with ideas and culture as mere 'reflexes' or 'appearance'. Hegemony points to a voluntaristic element in the structure of class domination foregrounding the active role of agents in legitimising forms of rule.
>
> (2000, p. 119)

These forms of resistance often take the form of struggles over culture, values and politics as various groups resist total incorporation within the dominant system. Within this complex dynamic, Gramsci adopts an anti-functionalist perspective, as it is this collective conflict, albeit conflict that is contained within hegemonic parameters, that helps shape society.

Gramsci saw the need for a revolutionary vanguard party to challenge the hegemony of the prevailing social order which he saw as being akin to Machiavelli's political treatise in *The Prince*. For Gramsci, *The Prince* could be read as 'a creation of concrete fantasy which acts on a dispersed and shattered people to arouse and organize its collective will' (quoted in Forgacs, 1999, p. 239). In the modern period it was not possible for the prince to be a real person, it had to be an organism,

> a complex element of society in which a collective will, which has already been recognised and has to some extent asserted itself in action, begins to take concrete form. History has already provided this organism, and it is the political party.
>
> (Ibid., p. 240)

Within Western Marxism, capitalism, with its expression via the ideological and cultural sphere embodied in the concept of hegemony, was seen as wielding the power previously held by the sovereign in terms of constituting subjects. As Clegg puts it,

> Hegemony becomes the metaphorical basis for constituting sovereign dominion.... Order, where it has been achieved, is secured by the sovereign power exerting dominion over the very ingredients of individual consciousness; the appetites, passions and especially the interests that these individuals have.
>
> (1989, p. 29)

Of importance, though, is that this power is negative,

> not simply because there are actors who negate, but because there are actors who, through no action of their own, can live their lives only as an unauthentic negation of their individual agency. Free to choose they may be, but

what they can choose from is already chosen: not specifically by anyone but by default and by virtue of what is discursively available for individuals to use to be or not to be actors in particular scenes.

(Ibid.)

In this respect the lack of political struggle, articulation or expression of grievance is not necessarily due to apathy but because the individual does not question his or her role in the prevailing social order. However, care has to be taken not to see subjects as mere puppets of hegemonic systems. In this respect, proponents of the theory of hegemony can, in their sovereign focused analysis of power, downplay the sovereignty of individual subjects who are seen as at the mercy of hegemonic ideologies and practices.

In *The German Ideology,* Marx and Engels (1970 [1846]) argue that 'the ruling ideas of every epoch are those of the ruling class' (p. 64). This idea has been taken by many radicals to explain the failure of the working class to seize its revolutionary role due to its members being unable to see the source of their oppression. However, for Clegg, Marx and Engels did not take such a systematic position around the incorporation of the working class into the capitalist system, their overall approach being more in line with Engels' position in *The Condition of the Working Class in England* (Engels, 1969 [1845]), in which he noted that the bourgeoisie has more in common with that of other nations than with the working class in its own country. Likewise, the working class speak their own dialects and have ideals and thoughts specific to their class and geographical position etc. In other words, rather than being bound to the ruling class by ideological hegemony, the working class are more akin to a foreign, unincorporated people.

Conclusion

The idea of false consciousness constitutes a problem for those who see human agency as the key attribute in challenging ruling ideologies and power relations. Implied in the concept is the notion that power is so all-embracing, so penetrating, that it has permeated the very subjectivity of individuals. So powerful is this sovereignty that those subject to it are unaware that they are in its embrace. In this respect it is difficult to envisage a way out as even at the point of our liberation we may in fact be further ensnared by the machinations of power.

Power that is not seen as such is seen as a greater threat to freedom than overt manifestations of power. So, for example, Žižek (2014) claims that the USA poses a more direct threat to the freedom of its population than China does to its. This is because whilst in a country such as China no one is under any illusions about the state restrictions on individual freedom, the limitations are clearly known. However, in the USA, there is the 'guarantee' of formal freedoms enshrined in law and the constitution, therefore most individuals experience their lives as free, unaware of the extent to which they are controlled by the state and its operational mechanisms. In this respect, the public exposure of the workings of power can alert us to the fact of our unfreedom, a reality that we were hitherto unaware of as we experience our lives as free.

There is, of course, a lot of truth in the fact that we are often unaware of the way power is working its way through society and ourselves. However, rather than this being seen as providing a compelling account of the need to embrace Kant's rallying call of Enlightenment humanism – 'Dare to know' – it can be used for anti-human purposes by those who would see us as mere dupes of ideology, genetics or biology. This is what Žižek infers by equating the ideologically controlled masses with rats. He describes the 2002 experiment whereby scientists attached a computer chip able to transmit signals directly to a rat's brain. This enabled the scientists to control the rat's movements by means of a remote control steering mechanism. In effect, the 'will' of a living animal was taken over by an external machine. The key question for Žižek is how the rat experienced its movements, movements that were not of its own volition but decided by an external power. How aware was it that its movements were subject to external control? Žižek believes that the answer to this question may indicate the difference between the 'free' citizens of Western liberal societies and their 'unfree' Chinese counterparts: 'the Chinese human rats are at least aware they are controlled, while we are the stupid rats strolling around unaware of how our movements are monitored' (Žižek, 2014, online). Speak for yourself Slavoj.

Those critical of the workings of the prevailing ideology argue for a need to see through its charade so that we can see the real workings of power and the reality of the systems that are oppressing us. From this perspective the goal was to help develop a 'false' consciousness into a more accurate form of consciousness. Ideology concealed the real, but what if there was no real to be exposed, merely further workings of power with no greater claim to the real than that which they replaced? This was the claim made by many writers, one of the most influential, for our purposes at least, being Michel Foucault. It is to his work that we now turn.

2   Power in postmodernity

Introduction

The Marxist conception of power, and concomitant notions of hegemony and ideology, attempted to provide a coherent (for its adherents at least) narrative of power. However, such interpretations were to be radically destabilised by the work of a variety of critics who have broadly been termed as postmodernists and/or poststructuralists, with perhaps the most influential of them being the French polymath, Michel Foucault. It would be difficult to underestimate the influence of Foucault's work on contemporary social and political thought. His ideas permeate much feminist and post-structural theory and have been incorporated into many sociological, psychological and philosophical schools of thought. Disciplines such as literary, film and textual criticism, feminist analysis, social history, penology and sexology have all been influenced by Foucault's work such as *Discipline and Punish*, *Madness and Civilisation*, *The History of Sexuality* and *The Order of Things*. Such a wide-ranging influence should not, however, be mistaken for an uncritical embracement of his ideas. On the contrary his work has been lauded, critically accepted and disparaged by various scholars, political activists and social theorists alike.

In this chapter I discuss both the strengths and limitations of Foucault's work, particularly with regard to his notions of power, governmentality and processes of subjectification. I wish to highlight some of the key themes within Foucault's work with particular reference to his analysis of power and of the debates that arose from them. Whilst much of this will be at a theoretical level, the intention is to highlight his influence on a range of theorists, activists and related social movements in order to situate understandings of power as they moved away from a focus on the structural, leviathan form of power and began to focus on the more micro aspects of power relations. As we will see in later chapters, this move has proved highly influential in the transition from notions of power to that of empowerment.

From sovereignty to governmentality

The situating of power with the monarch was, for Foucault, one of the central features of the transition from feudalism to modernity. In a period of great social turbulence, of conflict between various feudal groups, the monarch could present himself as arbiter between competing interest groups. Such sovereign power could be brutal and enacted directly on the body, as detailed by Foucault in *Discipline and Punish* which begins by detailing a 1757 order of the court in respect of 'Damiens the regicide' who was to be

> taken and conveyed in a cart, wearing nothing but a shirt, holding a torch of burning wax weighing two pounds; [then,] in the said cart, to the Place de Greve, where, on a scaffold that will be erected there, the flesh will be torn from his breasts, arms, thighs and calves with red-hot pincers, his right hand, holding the knife with which he committed the said parricide, burnt with sulphur, and, on those places where the flesh will be torn away, poured molten lead, boiling oil, burning resin, wax and sulphur melted together and then his body drawn and quartered by four horses and his limbs and body consumed by fire, reduced to ashes and his ashes thrown to the winds.[1]
>
> (Quoted in Foucault, 1991a [1977], p. 3)

There then follows a gruesome depiction of Damiens' public torturing and dismemberment. Foucault then goes on to describe the birth of the prison and the changing nature of both discipline and punishment from the medieval to the modern age. In the case of Damiens we can clearly see sovereign power being enacted on his body. However, the use of such power located within the sovereign (whether by right or law) began to be replaced by new forms of disciplinary power which were more diffuse and therefore more difficult to locate within any particular sovereign body.

Foucault's idea of governmentality entailed a genealogical analysis of what he termed the 'art of government'. His genealogical method sought to show both subjects and objects as historically contingent. In order to render apparently discrete practices intelligible his genealogy favoured the analysis of relations rather than a study of either objects or subjects as things in themselves. A genealogy is therefore a description and analysis of practices and facts interconnected with human experiences and modes of thought which he uses to analyse such things as madness, sexuality and crime.[2]

In charting the rise of the structures and practices of governance from the mid-sixteenth century, Foucault sought to detail the changing and widening forms of government that came into being with the development of the modern state. In this period,

> how to govern oneself, how to be governed, how to govern others, by whom the people will accept being governed, how to be the best possible governor – all these problems, in their multiplicity and intensity, seem to me characteristic of the sixteenth century.
>
> (Quoted in McNay, 1994, p. 113)

Arising from this, Foucault (1991a) argues that from the seventeenth and eighteenth centuries onwards there was an unquestionable technological increase in procedures for the productivity of power, of what he called a new 'economy' of power. There was a move towards state centralisation (in parallel with religious dissidence). Increasingly, the state and government was a topic for philosophical, political and public discussion alongside religious conflict and debate. What developed from this were 'procedures which allowed the effects of power to circulate in a manner at once continuous, uninterrupted, adapted, and "individualized" throughout the entire social body' (Foucault, 1980, p. 119). Social relations were increasingly subjected to an all-pervasive regime of normalising discipline. This new form of power contained highly specific procedural techniques, completely novel instruments, quite different apparatuses than those inherent within sovereign power. It is a form of power that is continually exercised by means of surveillance. This differs from monarchical or sovereign power.

In feudal days the exercise of power was more direct – for example, forcing the peasant to relinquish part of his product upon fear of punishment – but to a large extent his day to day life was not affected by the power of the sovereign. As Bauman notes, 'The sovereign power could remain distant from the body of the average producer, towering majestically at the far horizon of his life cycle … the customs and habits which ruled the daily life of the food suppliers were no concern of power' (1982, p. 40). The sovereign conception of power conceptualises power as being mostly absent except for when it is exercised, whereas for Foucault power is present even when it is seemingly absent. This confuses those who hold to a traditional sovereign view of power. Sovereign conceptions of power contend that it is episodic in nature and constituted mechanically, so that something has to be seen to have been done in order for it to be said that power has been exercised (Clegg, 1989).

This new form of government also differed from the earlier form in that previously the prince was in a position of singularity and transcendence in relation to his principality, within the later conception practices of government are multifarious and immanent in the state and society. McNay concisely points out the other key difference:

> in the juridical theory of sovereignty, a radical discontinuity is established and constantly redefined between the legitimate power of the prince and other 'illegitimate' forms of power. In contrast, a continuity is maintained between the different forms of power that compose the arts of government. There is an upward continuity in the sense that the person who governs the state well must first learn to govern himself correctly, and a downward continuity inasmuch, as when a state is well run, the head of a family will know how to look after his family, and individuals, in general, will behave correctly.
>
> (1994, p. 114)

This observation was, however, not enough for Foucault – a fixation on monarchical sovereignty, or in more recent times on state sovereignty, was still too narrow an interpretation of the concept of power. For him, it was essential to understand that power is not localised in the State apparatus because 'nothing in society will be changed if the mechanisms of power that function outside, below and alongside the State apparatuses, on a much more minute and everyday level, are also not changed' (Foucault, 1980, p. 60). Power, here, is relational, it is not a zero-sum game, and neither is it something that can be owned. Power is everywhere because it comes from everywhere. Power, 'insofar as it is permanent, repetitious, inert, and self-producing, is simply the over-all effect that emerges from all these mobilities' (Foucault, 1990, p. 93).

Foucault (1980) saw the mistake of the political left as being its focus on the State and its apparatus as the locale of power, although he also argued that there was just such a paucity in the analysis of power by both Left and Right during the post-Second World War period, with there being little attempt to adequately consider the means by which power was exercised 'concretely and in detail'. He emphasised the need to 'eschew the model of Leviathan in the study of power', to leave behind the limitations of analyses that focus on judicial sovereignty and State institutions, and to base the analysis of power on the subsidy of the techniques and tactics of domination. 'We must escape from the limited field of juridical sovereignty and State institutions, and instead base our analysis of power on the study of the techniques and tactics of domination' (p. 102). For Foucault, power was not something solely wielded by some unitary authority over passive individuals, on the contrary individuals 'are always in the position of simultaneously undergoing and exercising this power. They are not only its inert or consenting target; they are always also the elements of its articulation' (ibid., p. 98). Individuals are not merely nodal points to which power is applied but are vehicles of power. When power is exercised in such a way, through subtle mechanisms it 'cannot but evolve, organise and put into circulation a knowledge, or rather apparatuses of knowledge, which are not ideological constructs' (ibid., p. 102).

As we saw in the previous chapter, Hobbes contended that power should be invested in the body of the sovereign so as to prevent a war of all against all, a return to the 'state of nature'. In arguing for the need to 'cut off the King's head', in political theory terms, Foucault is seeking to reverse the mechanical analysis of power as being mechanical in the 'A has power over B' approach, but neither is his approach premised on the duality of agency and structure as in the works of Lukes (2005) or Giddens (1994). As Clegg (1989) puts it,

> Foucault seeks to show how relations of 'agency' and 'structure' have been constituted discursively,[3] how agency is denied to some and given to others, how structures could be said to have determined some things and not others. The focus is upon how certain forms of representation are constituted rather than upon the 'truth' or 'falsity' of the representations themselves.
>
> (p. 158, my footnote)

Instead of an abstract State wielding power over people, there was a need to see how power was dispersed throughout the social and literal body.

Sovereign power as traditionally conceived is negative. It prohibits behaviour that is proscribed by law. Foucault's conception of disciplinary power is, on the other hand, productive. As individuals are measured, examined, classified and objectified within discourse their bodily behaviour as well as their subjectivities are constituted. They find themselves the objects of expert knowledge. The productive element of the power/knowledge nexus contrasted with much of Western philosophical thinking, particularly its Platonic legacy that viewed power as being antithetical to knowledge in that it distorted our perceptions of reality. On the contrary, for Foucault 'there is no power relation without the correlative constitution of a field of power, nor any knowledge that does not constitute at the same time power relations' (1991a, p. 27). This was not the only radical departure of Foucault's line of reasoning. It followed from his argument that 'truth' could no longer be seen as something to be enlisted in the service of emancipation from oppression. Juridical power presupposes an implicit contract based on some shared conception of common interests that can be realised through the exercise of power. Therefore, workings of power that hinder the pursuit of such interests can be criticised for being illegitimate and oppressive. By contrast, disciplinary power is not based on such a social contract or shared conception of justice, and as a result 'resistance can no longer be understood on the normative model of emancipation from unjust social and political relations (Cronin, 1996, p. 59).

In calling into question 'truth' as being merely a product of power/knowledge, there being no human essence, Foucault's 'radical decentering of the knowing and willing subject is to sever the connection between resistance and normative conceptions of truth and justice, at least as these are traditionally understood' (ibid). Of importance is that in this conceptualisation there is no objective standpoint outwith relations of power, and as such no way to ascertain 'truth'. What is held to be 'truth' at any given point is merely the *effects of truth* established via dominant discourses.

It is important to acknowledge the period in which Foucault was developing his work. He was undoubtedly influenced by the social and political unrest of the 1960s, a period in which existing social and political relations were being challenged by various social actors. In this changing and contested climate Foucault concluded that a new form of analysis of power was necessary: 'From all these different experiences, including my own, there emerged only one word, like a message written in invisible ink, ready to appear on the page when the right chemical is added; and the word is power' (1991b, pp. 145–146, emphasis in original).

In arguing that we needed to look at the exercise of power within and through the social body rather than as something directly imposed from above, Foucault argued that modernity was characterised by two concepts of power – 'disciplinary power' and 'bio-power' – which were contrasted with sovereign power. Disciplinary power is concerned with the control of particular individuals or groups whereas biopower refers to the way power subjugates the general population. For example, in his work on sexuality Foucault argued that far from being an age of sexual repression, the concern with repression conversely led to an obsession with sex, there emerging a plethora of theoretical writings, political and public discussions over what is and is not normal sexual behaviour, and also in such things as architectural design where plans for such things as schools would have to detail separate toilets and sleeping areas for boys and girls. The very desire to regulate sexuality led to a fixation with it. Biopower then refers to discourses that regulate and limit behaviours and desires, with the fields of social work, medicine and psychiatry being exemplars of this process as they institutionalise and regulate that which is said to deviate from the normal. However, the true power of biopower lies in processes whereby such established meanings get incorporated into our everyday ways of thinking and behaving. As such, power is productive, it helps produce our very subjectivity. In this respect, the subject of power is not passive, actors play a part in the construction of the self via available forms of meaning. As McLaughlin puts it:

> The socially produced and disciplined subject is not a determined and passive subject. Individuals are actively involved in the processes of subjectification that discipline them. The issue is why and how 'a human being turns him – or herself into a subject' (Foucault, 1982, p. 208)? In part the answer is that when we adopt available subject positions, as well as being disciplined we also adopt a positive sense of self that is able to participate in the world. Individuality may be fictional and follow templates, but we have agency in the creative part we play in making that individual unique to us.
>
> (2003, p. 119)

Far from seeing new 'social' and 'scientific' disciplines as benign, he shows how the emergence of new professions such as medicine, law, psychiatry and social work developed new forms of codifying, regulating and disciplining bodies. For example, the fear of being classified as 'mad' had the effect of making people regulate and discipline their own bodies, to behave in a 'respectable' socially acceptable way. A similar sentiment was expressed by the 'anti-psychiatrist' David Cooper who argued that the main purpose of psychiatry was not to cure madness. According to him,

> Psychiatric treatment is often ridiculed in terms of its failure [to cure madness] but this is most unjust. If one is to speak truly of the failure of psychiatric treatment one must be prepared to see that its failure resides most precisely in its success. This treatment either in its official or unofficial guise (non-medical therapeutic conditioning) usually succeeds in producing a requisite conformism either on the level of the chronic back ward or on the (higher or lower) level of the all-commanding captain of industry.
>
> (Cooper, 1967, p. 17)

In this sense, Marxist analyses that focused on the state, economy and class relations are seen as being too reductionist to allow us to gain a detailed picture of the workings of power. Instead of such a top-down analysis an ascending analysis of power was necessary. As McNay summarises it,

> if power generates a multiplicity of effects, then it is only possible to discern these effects by analysing power from below, at its most precise points of operation – a microphysics of power. The human body is the most specific point at which the micro strategies of power can be observed. It is a microphysical analysis of the operations of power upon the body that yields the notion of 'disciplinary' or 'bio' power explored in detail in *Discipline and Punish*.
>
> (1994, p. 91)

We are constantly being watched over and monitored, the objects of a disciplinary gaze.

The power of the gaze

The Panoptican was a design by Jeremy Bentham for the 'perfect prison'. In the centre was the central tower with passageways leading out to cells that formed a circle around the centre. The guard in the centre of the tower could observe all the prisoners, but crucially they could not see the guard. The key idea was that the gaze of the guard was always felt by the prisoners; even if not being literally observed, the fact that they could be was enough to instil obedience in them. In other words, the power of the gaze instils self-surveillance in those subject to it. It is a form of power which has

> no need for arms, physical violence, material constraints. Just a gaze. An inspecting gaze, a gaze which each individual under its weight will end by interiorising to the point that he is his own observer, each individual thus exercising this surveillance over, and against himself.
>
> (Foucault, 1980, p. 155)

The attraction of Foucault's theories for feminism is clear to see given his focus on the family and its governance and on the more micro aspects of power relations. He was, in effect, warning them, and structural Marxists influenced by Althusser, that by placing too much emphasis on the power of the State they risked ignoring or downplaying the capillaries of power that permeate the social system and all social relations. Such disciplinary or biopower works through, not on, bodies, embedding itself in the behaviour and unconscious of the subject. Bartky gives the following example of the power of the male gaze on female behaviour:

> The woman who checks her make-up half a dozen times a day to see if her foundation has caked or her mascara has run, who worries that the wind or rain may spoil her hairdo, who looks frequently to see if her stockings have bagged at the ankle, or who, feeling fat, monitors everything she eats, has become, just as surely as the inmate of the Panoptican, a self-policing

subject, a self committed to a relentless surveillance. This self-surveillance is a form of obedience to patriarchy.

(1990, p. 80)

That Foucault's theories have been highly influential does not mean that they have been met with universal approval, more a critical appraisal that seeks to modify and improve them. His work was criticised within feminist circles for being gender blind and therefore failing to appreciate the centrality of gender to the operation and development of modern concepts of subjectivity. Janice McLaughlin summarises the strengths and weaknesses of Foucault for feminism as being ultimately useful because they encourage us to consider

> sources of discipline in society and industrial relations; women's incorpora-tion of surveillance, the role of discourses in the production of identity; the politics of knowledge and claims to truth; resistant practices within everyday relations. However, using some of his ideas requires an approach ready to move beyond his lack of interest in important areas, including: gender; polit-ical engagement, economic inequality [and] actions as well as discourses.
>
> (McLaughin, 2003, p. 130)

Sawicki (1991) argues that we can take on board the insights Foucault gives, but that strategies for emancipation have to be achieved without him. The problem is that in claiming that the subject is a false concept, Foucault has also reduced the concept of subjectivity. The weight of power is too great to be challenged by the mere 'objects' of history. Hartsock similarly argues that

> Rather than getting rid of subjectivity or notions of the subject, as Foucault does, and substituting his notion of the individual as an effect of power rela-tions, we need to engage in the historical, political, and theoretical process of constituting ourselves as subjects as well as objects.
>
> (1998, p. 221)

The suggestion that the critique of the subject could itself be a male, patriarchal inspired conspiracy against feminist demands for equality is implied by Hartsock when she writes

> Why is it that just at the moment when so many of us who have been silenced begin to demand the right to name ourselves, to act as subjects rather than objects of history, that just then the concept of subjecthood becomes problematic? Just when we are forming our own theories about the world, uncertainty emerges about whether the world can be theorized. Just when we are talking about the changes we want, ideas of progress and the possibility of systematically and rationally organizing human society become dubious and suspect.
>
> (1998, p. 210)

Whilst Hartsock's reasoning is unconvincing in terms of cause and effect, she does alert us to the possibility that critiques of power by oppressed groups can be manipulated and distorted to give outcomes that were not those intended by the original advocates. The evacuation of the subject from theoretical and political life does have consequences for personal and political life, and later chapters of the thesis will focus on specific aspects of this within the rise and institutionalisation of empowerment.

This idea that the discursively constituted subject lacks agency is rejected by many feminists. For example, Butler (2006 [1990]) argues that, 'Construction is not opposed to agency; it is the necessary scene of agency' (p. 147), whilst Sawicki suggests that feminists have mistaken social constructionism for determinism due to them being trapped in the binary logic of Western thought,

> We have mistaken the self for a thing because of our participation in Cartesian and ultimately Hegelian discursive traditions, which postulate a subject/ object dichotomy and identify liberation with the epistemological project of the subject's discovery of itself in the objective world.
>
> (1991, p. 299)

The subject in the Foucaultian sense is not separate or at one end of a subject/ object dichotomy but rather is shaped by discursive and regulatory practices. The individual is not a sovereign subject but is 'itself only a parody: it is plural; countless spirits dispute its possession; numerous sections intersect and compete' (Foucault, 1991c, p. 94). The problem with such a reading is that it renders the subject as nothing more than a localised point of intersection. Furthermore, this intersection is one in which the subject is in continual conflict with others due to the omnipresence of power. Whilst Foucault is of the belief that power generates resistance, the conflict is an ongoing and directionless one in which there is no unifying force or agent; instead, and apparently ad infinitum, we are in constant combat. We are in danger of a return to the model of the individual that Hobbes proposed as existing in a state of war, of all against all, but where the Leviathan is replaced not by a Hegelian synthesis but a negative dialectics that further disassembles the subject.

However, for some feminists he went too far in downplaying the role of the social structure on the lives of women. For feminists whose critique focused on structural patriarchy, 'the call to move away from analyses of material and economic power relations appears to deny feminism the ability to discuss the systematic nature of women's oppression' (McLaughlin, 2003, p. 132). His focus on the body and his refusal of a normative framework in which a collective analysis could be articulated leads to the charge that his focus on the individual, a key feature of feminism as a beginning, goes no further and becomes mere individualism (McNay, 1994).

In addition, Foucault has been criticised for failing to account for the way that individual subjectivity is internalised via interpretation and evaluation, with the consequence that there is a danger of the subject being reduced to a mere reflex of bodily habits induced by external stimuli (Cronin, 1996). Foucault (1983) was not unaware of the problematic consequences of decentring the subject to such an extent that the subject is lost altogether, arguing that power is exercised over an agent and that 'power is exercised only over free subjects, and only insofar as they are free' (p. 221), although in much of his writing this free subject is difficult to discern.

The attention given to biopower as the working through of political power relations also led to a focus on strategies to subvert and overcome them. A recent example of this occurred in 2014, when a group of women used social media to post pictures of their unshaved legs in protest against the social pressure on women to have them shaved, waxed and smooth (Murphy, 2014), although how progressive the blurring of the personal and political in such a way threatens the status quo in any fundamental way is open to question. As we will see in the next chapter, such posting of an individual photo on social media is a far cry from the more radical, collective roots of the earlier feminists.

Foucault also challenged Weberian analyses that focused on the functional stratification of spheres of social action and of how they were consolidated within the institutions of the modern state, and Marxist conceptions that saw modernisation as entailing the unfolding of the internal dynamic inherent within a capitalist economic social system. However, he does share some common ground with Weber, in that he is seeking 'clarity about our historical nightmare' or as Weber himself put it, the 'mighty cosmos of the modern economic order ... the iron cage [in which] specialists without spirit, sensualists without heart, [are] caught in the delusion that [they] have achieved a level of development never before attained by mankind' (Rabinow, 1991, pp. 26–27).

Both Weber and Foucault offer a pessimistic account of their society. Whilst often labelled a conservative, Weber's critiques of existing capitalism and its effects on the individual are trenchant, and for his part, Foucault, seen as aligned with the Left, is opposed to the French Marxist tradition and the 'real existing socialism' of the period in which he was writing. For Rabinow,

> What both Weber and Foucault proffer – in a pessimistic and dour mode in Weber's case, and an elusive and joyous one in Foucault's – is a heroic refusal to sentimentalize the past in any way or to shirk the necessity of facing the future as dangerous but open. Both have committed their lives to a scrupulous, if unorthodox, forging of intellectual tools for the analysis of modern rationality, social and economic organization and subjectivity. Both see a form of critical historicism as the only road to preserving reason and the obligation – differently understood by Weber and Foucault – to forge an ascetic ethic of scientific and political responsibility as the highest duty of the mature intellectual.
>
> (Ibid., p. 27)

In referring to Foucault's work as joyous, Rabinow is in a minority as often Foucault is read as giving a pessimistic account of modern power relations and the ordeal of the subject. If, as Foucault argues, power 'is co-extensive with the social body; there are no spaces of primal liberty between the meshes of its network' (1980, p. 142), then we are trapped within a web of power from which there is seemingly no prospect of liberation. All the 'truths' of a given society are particular to it, reflective of the types of discourse that it accepts as legitimate.

> 'Truth' is to be understood as a system of ordered procedures for the production, regulation, distribution, circulation and operation of statements. 'Truth' is linked in a circular relation with systems of power which produce and sustain it, and to effects of power which it induces and which extend it. A 'regime' of truth'.
>
> (Foucault, 1980, p. 133)

In other words there was no 'grand narrative'. In some respects Foucault's work shares some assumptions with the Frankfurt School and Habermas:

> Both unmask the Cartesian Subject, understood as a fixed and universal foundation prior to experience.... Both eschew the notion that knowledge is disinterested contemplation of a pre-given object; instead, given the priority of material practice, they assume that knower and knowable mutually constitute one another as meaningful identities. Finally, by *reflecting* on their own practical genealogy, both critiques seek to enlighten individuals about the social conditions under which their identities, needs and interests are historically constituted.
>
> (Ingram, 1994, p. 218, emphasis in original)

Foucault sought to show that there was no transcendental subject nor natural object, rather both subjects and objects were co-emergent and constituted through a discourse that preceded them both. What we know and how we know it is grounded by our experiences, which in turn are governed by our particular life circumstances, and are historically and geographically situated. Our subjectivity therefore is contingent, not universal and timeless, nor unfolding teleologically towards its historical destiny. Foucault attempted to show how practices and beliefs, such as attitudes to homosexuality, madness and punishment were shaped by many factors and not due to some abstract universal notions of essentialism or reason.

Within the feminist movement, with its critique of aspects of Enlightenment universalism and humanism justifying women's oppression, it is unsurprising that Foucault's work was influential. However, some feminists were criticised for adopting universal and absolutist categories of their own. According to Sawicki,

> White, middle class feminists often unwittingly embraced universal categories and concepts of femininity that erase differences among women

(differences of race, class, sexual orientation, ethnicity, religion, *and so on*) in ways that parallel their own erasure within androcentric humanisms). [This is] despite the fact that there are good reasons to believe that 'femininity' itself is a masculinist construction, many feminists are reluctant to abandon appeals to absolute foundations – to some essential, liberatory subject rooted in 'women's experience' (or nature) – as a starting point for an emancipatory theory.

(1991, p. 289, my emphasis)

This argument raises issues around identity politics such as to what extent can an identity be useful for political purposes if by its nature it excludes others. However, as the words 'and so on' imply, the notion of difference can be expanded to include almost any identity or experience; after all, every individual is unique. Holding on to an inclusive collective experience, without it collapsing into fragmentation is an inherent problem for those who advocate the politics of identity and difference. As we will see in Chapter 3, there is a growing trend to try to go beyond some of these problems by those who advocate an intersectional approach to identity, power and difference.

Power and resistance

From a Foucauldian perspective, there is no rational autonomous agent outside the machinations of power. If power is all pervasive, then there can be no autonomous subject free from its effects. Also, if power is ubiquitous can there be any points of resistance to its workings? In answer to such criticisms, Foucault gave this oft-quoted reply: 'Where there is power, there is resistance, and yet, or rather consequently, this resistance is never in a position of exteriority in relation to power' (1990, p. 95).

Despite this partial concession to agentic resistance Foucault's objects of analysis are just that, objects as opposed to social actors. So, whilst he prioritised questions of domination and discipline, he failed to adequately address the question of agency and resistance in his analysis of power. As Allen has noted, Foucault

never offers a detailed account of resistance as an empirical phenomenon in any of his genealogical analyses. The only social actors in these works are dominating agents; there is no discussion of the strategies employed by madmen, delinquents, schoolchildren, perverts, or 'hysterical' women to modify or contest the disciplinary or bio-power exercised over them.

(1999, p. 54)

In seeing the subject as an effect of technologies of the self, Foucault has been accused of positing a crude form of behaviourism, the self a mere product of constant conditioning (Honneth, 1991). Indeed, it is precisely the undermining of the rational, agentic self that shows, I would contend, why it is necessary to understand Foucault's work, as this aspect of it, as we shall see in later chapters, underpins much of contemporary politics.

Where Foucault does offer some strategies of resistance is in terms of self-refusal:

> Maybe the target nowadays is not to discover what we are but to refuse what we are.... The conclusion would be that the political, ethical, social, philosophical problem of our days is not to try to liberate the individual from the state, and from the state's institutions, but to liberate us both from the state and from the type of individualization which is linked to the state. We have to promote new forms of subjectivity through refusal of this kind of individuality which has been imposed on us for several centuries.
>
> (Foucault, 1982, p. 785)

Foucault is less forthcoming in how we can go about this endeavour, and this failure to provide any answers as to how resistance to domination can be possible is something for which he has often been criticised. However, negative criticism, a diagnosis without a prognosis, is useful in and of itself, as in order to resist oppression we must be aware of the ways in which we are being oppressed, and why should we look to Foucault to lead us to the promised land, in doing so we can absolve ourselves of the responsibility of forging our own future both individually and collectively. In any event, as Sawicki notes:

> Through the analysis, description and criticism of existing power/knowledge relations Foucault hoped to create the space necessary for resistance, for taking advantage of what he referred to as the 'tactical polyvalence' of discourses and practices, and for developing oppositional strategies and new forms of experience.
>
> (1991, p. 294)

Nevertheless, Foucault's locating of power in terms of impersonal relations of force and strategies, rather than to the individual or groups, whilst often alerting us to the former having their own histories that are not totally reducible to the intentionality of individuals or groups, and can have unintended consequences, is also problematic. Echoing Charles Taylor, Cronin notes that a strategy is, in essence, connected with agency and social practice, in that whilst 'cases where individual or collective actions have unintended consequences provide us with examples of purposefulness that cannot be reduced to the conscious motives, choices, or decisions of individuals or groups' (1996, p. 60) nevertheless, it is still possible to claim that such consequences exhibit considered and intentional patterns if we are able to relate them to the conscious motivations of identifiable social agents.

Foucault's critique of subject-centred notions of power have also been criticised for rendering it impossible to identify any social location of the exercise of, or resistance to, power and that his monolithic 'disciplinary society' fails to account for the diverse forms of power at work in modern societies (Cronin, 1996). To avoid getting caught in such intellectual quicksand several look to the work of another French theorist, Pierre Bourdieu, in particular his work on symbolic power and the interaction between field and habitus (e.g. McNay, 1994). The work of Foucault and Bourdieu share much in common. Each was concerned with providing a critique of subject-centred analyses of power which they do with often penetrating insights into the workings of modern institutions and societal interactions.

Bourdieu's conception of power and bodily discipline differs from Foucault's in an important way, and one that allows us to critically understand the operations of state power in a more Marxist sense without overly focusing on state apparatuses, as, say Althusser has been criticised for, at the expense of seeking to show the workings of power in more micro forms of social interaction. It is important to recall that Foucault's disciplinary techniques of surveillance, measurement, classification and normalisation were developed within closed institutions such as the prison and asylum and he then applied this model to wider society. They are novel techniques of objectification and productive of subjectivity. In Bourdieusian terms we may say that Foucault is trying to explain the internalisation of the habitus. However, as Cronin (1996) points out, for Bourdieu, the inculcation of the habitus is not due to new techniques of surveillance and normalisation, but arises from everyday injunctions concerning posture, manners, 'correct' pronunciation, etc., 'by which parents instil into their children behavioural dispositions and schemes of perception and evaluation, which are subsequently reinforced by the education system' (Cronin, 1996, p. 73). Therefore, modern forms of power should not be seen as the result of the emergence of new technologies for disciplining bodies, but of 'the normalization, objectification and formalization of *practices* through codification, which lead to new forms of symbolic power connected with the institutions of the modern state' (ibid., emphasis in original).

However, the strategic model of social action developed by Bourdieu still remains too narrow in that it does not allow the possibility of autonomous agency, something that renders it insufficient as a way of formulating emancipatory political praxis. For such emancipatory potential to be realised, 'the theory of symbolic power must be supplemented by a normative conception of practical reason' (ibid., p. 55).

In reply to criticisms that his analysis leaves little scope for human agency, with individuals seemingly trapped in a matrix of power, Foucault does acknowledge that 'power is only exercised over free subjects, and only insofar as they are free. By this we mean individual or collective subjects who are faced with a field of possibilities in which several ways of behaving, several reactions and diverse comportments may be realized' (1982, p. 790). Nevertheless, even where his work has met with general, if qualified, approval, this problem of agentic resistance remains paramount.

Conclusion

Foucault in many ways changed the terms of the debate over power even though he rarely specified or pinned down 'power', instead referring to it more in terms of it being 'a practice', associated with 'discipline' and the 'drilling' of bodies, via medical, psychiatric or social work discourse and related techniques. In many respects Foucault places 'the subject' with 'the body' as that which is to be analysed. Nevertheless, as we have seen, he also found himself accused of focusing too much on institutions of power that were monolithic, unidirectional and able to inflict harm on docile and powerless subjects. This approach is more evident in work such as *Discipline and Punish* than it is in his later work, such as *History of Sexuality*, where he acknowledged the fluidity and contingent nature of power relations and, crucially, the idea that resistance always exists where there is power.

Perhaps we can have it both ways; we can take on board many of Foucault's insights without being trapped in a subjectless world where we are mere intersections of a power/knowledge nexus. It is surely possible to view the ideal of the sovereign subject as just that, an ideal, whilst simultaneously holding on to the possibility of moving forward towards increased knowledge and autonomy. Truth with a capital 'T' may be like the carrot before the donkey in that it is always just ahead of us, but this does not negate the need to reach out and travel along the road to enlightenment.

It is also possible to acknowledge the power of many to define a behaviour, an action, an attribute as sick, deviant or unnatural, and in so doing make the individuals so defined as liable to be treated in certain ways, for example, medical treatment or hospitalisation for those labelled 'mad', compulsion or imprisonment for those deemed deviant or criminal. In doing so we can adopt an approach that does not negate either the potential for good that professionals can achieve nor downplay the distress caused to individuals and society by mental distress and criminality.

So, whilst there are many valid criticisms of Foucault, his idea that what can be presented as progressive social and/or scientific developments may disguise underlying forces of subjectification and objectification is worth holding onto. Indeed, as we shall see in later chapters, aspects of his analyses can illuminate the workings of power as they operate via the discourse of empowerment and through the bodies of those ostensibly being 'empowered'.

Notes

1 Damiens stabbed King Louis XV of France on 5 January, 1757. The king survived, suffering only a light wound and Damiens was apprehended immediately. The charge of parricide was because the king was seen as the father of his subjects.
2 The utilisation of the term 'genealogy' clearly shows the influence of, if not strict adherence to, the work of Nietzsche on Foucault. In *Power/Knowledge* he writes:

> The only valid tribute to a thought such as Nietzsche's is precisely to use it, to deform it, to make it groan and protest. And if commentators then say that I am being faithful or unfaithful to Nietzsche, that is of absolutely no importance.
>
> (Foucault, 1980, pp. 53–54)

3 Foucault distinguishes discourse from ideology in that discourse does not conceal something 'real' ostensibly concealed due to the workings of ideology.

3   From power to empowerment

Introduction

The previous two chapters have guided us through some of the complexities of the concept of power, focusing on early sociological explanations through to the more postmodern formulations of the workings of power. This was necessary in order for us to have a baseline understanding of the term to then try and locate the dynamics behind the rise, meaning and implications of the relatively new concept of empowerment.

To get an understanding of the way that the meaning of empowerment has changed over time it is necessary to look at how it was conceptualised in the past. To do so, this chapter will focus on the way social groups articulated their concerns in the pursuit of personal and political change, with a particular focus on black feminist and disability/deaf activists' attempts to understand and change their circumstances. From such work emerged the rise of intersectional thinking as a way to understand, explain and challenge interlinked forms of oppression. These examples are used to highlight two key issues: first, the way that, in its earlier manifestations, empowerment was often expressed in the language of identity-based social movements and contained within it a radical component; and, second, to show the influence of social constructionist and anti-essentialist theoretical perspectives as utilised in the political sphere.

Despite the radical roots of such attempts at empowerment there are some inherent tensions within identity/intersectional politics that have been exacerbated in the contemporary period as it has influenced, and in turn been influenced by, a 'vulnerability zeitgeist' (Brown, 2015), a period in which there has been a loss of a sense of a social anchor with which to locate ourselves and make sense of our difficulties. The chapter concludes by arguing that the radical fervour of the early manifestations of empowerment has waned as the term has become institutionalised within political, health and social welfare discourse and practice, a position that is then developed further in subsequent chapters.

The radical roots of empowerment

One of the earliest attempts at defining empowerment was in relation to social work with Black communities in the USA, where Solomon (1976) defined it as 'a process whereby persons who belong to a stigmatized social category throughout their lives can be assisted to develop and increase skills in the exercise of interpersonal influence and performance of valued social roles' (p. 6). Whilst this can be read as a more micropolitical manifestation of empowerment, others within the Black community adopted the term for more radical political purposes. One key text from this perspective is Patricia Hill Collins' *Black Feminist Thought: Knowledge, Consciousness, and the Politics of Empowerment* (Hill Collins, 1990). In this book Hill Collins states that she wants to 'find a voice' and 'replace the external definitions of my life forwarded by dominant groups with my own self-defined standpoint' (pp. xi–xii). However, the voice she was seeking to liberate was not a solely internal subjective one, but one that is 'both individual and collective, personal and political, one reflecting the intersection of my unique biography with the larger meaning of my historical times' (p. xii). In developing Black Feminist thought the ideas and experiences of African-American women were to be the focus of analysis.

Hill Collins was alert to the dangers of presenting Black Feminist thought as something without contradictions, frictions and inconsistencies. However, she downplays these issues, and in an echo of Spivak's (1987) notion of 'strategic essentialism', sees the need to portray it as overly coherent at the specific historical period in which she was writing. In this sense the book can be seen as attempting to instigate an intellectual tradition alongside social and political struggle that could, albeit later in the process, have the complexities and contradictions within it highlighted, discussed and hopefully resolved.

In attempting to raise the voices of black women it is noted that there exists a historical tradition of black women's intellectual thought but that such knowledge has been erased from history, their experiences and ideas silenced, largely suppressed and forgotten. Such a process is not accidental. Drawing on the work of writers such as Fanon (1963) and Friere (1970) the suppression of the knowledge produced by subordinate groups is seen as being part of the system of control that allows dominant groups to maintain their rule, in part because the oppressed are liable to internalise the ideological justifications for their low social status.

The suppression of black women's ideas is not seen as solely the result of white male hegemony; white feminist organisations were also charged with ignoring or marginalising black women intellectuals and activists. So too were their black male counterparts. For example, the Black Feminist activist, Pauli Murray, noted that the *Journal of Negro History* contained only five articles that focused exclusively on black women between its inception in 1916 and 1970, although such a situation began to be addressed during the 1970s and 1980s (cited in Hill Collins, 1990).

In developing her theory of the development of awareness of, and resistance to, oppression, Hill Collins argues that the knowledge gained from their experiences as subjugated beings at the intersection of race, gender and class oppression 'provides the stimulus for crafting and passing on the subjugated knowledge of a Black women's culture of resistance' (1990, p. 10). Here, she highlights the contradictions between the prevailing ideology of womanhood and the lived experience of black women, asking, 'If women are allegedly passive and fragile, then why are Black women treated as "mules" and assigned heavy cleaning chores?' She invokes Sojourner Truth's famous 1851 'Ain't I a Woman?' speech:

> That man over there says that women need to be helped into carriages, and lifted over ditches, and to have the best place everywhere. Nobody ever helps me into carriages, or over mud-puddles, or gives me any best place! And ain't I a woman? Look at me! Look at my arm! I have ploughed and planted, and gathered into barns, and no man could head me! And ain't I a woman? I could work as much and eat as much as a man – when I could get it – and bear the lash as well! And ain't I a woman? I have borne five children, and seen most all sold off to slavery, and when I cried out with my mother's grief, none but Jesus heard me! And ain't I a woman?
>
> (Quoted in Hill Collins, 1990, p. 14)

It is important to note that for some the struggle for black female emancipation was part of a wider struggle for human dignity and empowerment that was at heart a humanist, universalising, project. Speaking in 1893, Anna Julia Cooper pointed out that

> We [black women] take our stand on the solidarity of humanity, the oneness of life, and the unnaturalness and injustice of all special favouritisms, whether of sex, race, country or condition' and not until the pursuit of happiness is conceded to be inalienable to all; not till then is woman's lesson taught and woman's cause won – not the white woman's nor the black woman's, not the red woman's but the cause of every man and of every woman who has writhed silently under a mighty wrong.
>
> (Quoted in Hill Collins, 1990, p. 37)

Regardless of the particular political solutions that are proposed in specific situations or historical contexts, at heart such political action to achieve social transformation is seen 'as a *means* for human empowerment rather than ends in and of themselves' (ibid., emphasis in original).

Of course, Black Feminist activists were not the only ones railing against the status quo, many other groups were also doing so, and one that challenged much of the prevailing consensus was around disability in general (e.g. Morris, 1991; Oliver, 1996), and deafness in particular. This latter issue is worth considering in some more detail to add weight to my 'radical roots of empowerment' argument.

From deaf to Deaf

The Deaf community's struggle for social equality also highlights the way in which empowerment was seen as something to be fought for, as a product of struggle against the perceived inequitable treatment of deaf people by the 'normal' hearing world. Whilst having certain parallels with the disability movement in terms of challenging normative frameworks of normal and abnormal, there is one crucial difference. The physical disability movement draws a distinction between impairment and disability, the former being, for example, the loss of a limb, the latter being the problems caused when the impairment meets a social environment not organised around the impairment. From this perspective, a wheelchair user's mobility problems would be seen as due more to a lack of accessible transport than individual impairment. However, the Deaf (with a capital D) community does not see deafness as constituting a disability at all. On the contrary, to be deaf is to belong to a cultural and linguistic minority. From this perspective, measures to 'cure' deafness can be viewed as tantamount to genocide, the deliberate elimination of a devalued minority group.

In her history of the Deaf community Jankowski (1997) details how the group emerged, paradoxically, as a result of the segregation of deaf people from the wider community. Unwelcome in the public sphere and placed in residential schools or asylums outside mainstream society, they used their enforced confinement to develop a 'class' or 'common community'. As she puts it, 'the evolution of a separate sphere for Deaf people enabled them to build a community on their own terms' (p. 44). However, this creation of a separate sphere is neither natural nor unavoidable as the example of Martha's Vineyard illustrates.

Martha's Vineyard is an island to the south of Boston, Massachusetts in the USA where hereditary deafness used to be fairly common within the community. What is interesting though is that deaf individuals were fully included in the life of the community, and in contrast to eugenicist policies pursued elsewhere, they were free to marry deaf or hearing persons. Historical records indicate that this acceptance of deaf people had been going on for more than three centuries (Groce, 1993). Groce's research, which included interviews with residents of Martha's Vineyard, details a community in which deafness was accepted, with some interviewees puzzled by her, or indeed the mainland press's, interest in the subject; to them deafness was unremarkable, a normal part of community life. The inability to hear simply had no bearing on the deaf person's status within the community.

As one respondent said:

> The only time I ever thought about it was when I read an article in the Boston paper. I thought it was so funny that they should write about it in the paper.... It struck me funny that they should have an article, because to me, you know, it was something very ordinary and I used to think, wasn't it funny that a Boston paper would be interested in it.
>
> (Quoted in Groce, 1993, p. 145)

Questions as to why there was such a high incidence of deafness on the island tended only to arise for people after they had visited the mainland when they realised that other communities did not have any significant number of deaf inhabitants. The example of Martha's Vineyard is often held up as a key factor in the social construction of disability; after all, if deaf people could be fully integrated into society there, why could they not be fully integrated elsewhere. In other words, there was nothing essential about deafness that automatically led to deaf people being marginalised or medicalised.

As we have noted, ideology, communicated through rhetoric, is considered a crucial aspect in the way social movements challenge power. For Jankowski (1997), 'a social movement that transforms ideology into rhetoric has the potential to acquire power. This process of *acquiring* power transforms feelings of powerlessness into feelings of empowerment' (p. 3, my emphasis). Of importance here is the focus on acquiring, not being given, power. The marginalised group, in this instance the Deaf community, struggles to alter the distribution of power between itself and the hearing world. The influence of Foucault is clear as there is a pivotal focus given to the role of discourse in the construction of social reality; as such it can both create and sustain power, but, crucially, it can also challenge and subvert it.

For Alexander Graham Bell, deafness was something he would prefer to see eradicated or at least contained, as for him it represented 'a great calamity to the world' and to allow it to grow would lead to the spread of 'a defective race of human beings' (quoted in Jankowski, 1997, p. 53). Bell favoured the dismantling of group separatism within specialist schools for deaf children in favour of integrating them into mainstream schooling, preferably one per mainstream classroom. He saw no place for deaf teachers as they were not considered conducive to the goal of the encouragement of speech-reading.

In discussing the way the Deaf community challenged its portrayal and treatment by the hearing world, Jankowski (1997) notes how the community 'ferociously battled', calling for an end to what they saw as the domination, condemnation and correction of deaf people, and of how they refused to sit passively and accept the destruction of their community that they saw as being threatened by polices of oralism and integration.

The importance of the development of sign language for the Deaf community cannot be underestimated. Speech is the primary form of human communication, and the ability to communicate with our fellow humans is seen as a key aspect of our humanity. Prior to the development of sign language it was not uncommon for deaf people to be viewed as more beast than human. Sign language allowed deaf people to articulate their thoughts, to communicate with each other and the hearing world, to show that they were human, not beasts. For the British deaf activist Paddy Ladd, founder of the National Union for the Deaf in 1976 and one time national administrator of the British Deaf Association, it was learning British Sign Language at the age of 22 that gave him entry into the Deaf community. Ladd campaigned to have television programmes made that addressed issues of concern to deaf people and became the first deaf presenter on the BBC television programme *See Hear* (Prasad, 2003).

With sign language seen as a central, if not the central, aspect of deaf identity, it follows that anything that threatens its legitimacy and existence necessitates a robust response. In presenting sign language as a means of communication on a par with spoken language, as a different but equally valid method of communication, anything that threatened it also threatened the community itself; presented as the defining feature of a linguistic and cultural minority, sign language had to be defended at any cost.

In addition, medical and technological advances were perceived as a direct threat to the existence of the Deaf community. In this respect the development of hearing aids and cochlear implants which may allow deaf people to gain some hearing are not heralded as a positive development, but on the contrary are said to 'symbolize age-old dominant practices to convert Deaf people into hearing people' (Jankowski, 1997, p. 142). Some go further and see such practices as akin to genocide similar to the Nazi Holocaust, with this Final Solution being directed at the Deaf rather than Jewish community (Solomon, 1994, p. 65). The Nazi parallel is also invoked in relation to the tendency to trial cochlear implants on the young: 'Like the Nazis, they seem to enjoy experimenting on little children' (ibid.).

Oralist polices are accused of causing mental health problems for deaf children and should be categorised as a form of child abuse (Ladd, 2003). Mather and Mitchell (1994) use the term 'communication abuse', which they describe as the 'abuse of a child through the refusal of a care-giver or teacher to provide a language, the provision of an inadequate language, or the failure to provide full access to communication' (p. 12). The use of such discourse is held to be a radical call in that it rejects minimal accommodation and demands full participation and integration into society (Jankowski, 1997), although from the vantage point of today it could also be seen as an early example of a social movement using children to emphasise a moral or political claim, something that is increasingly common in the current period (McLaughlin, 2015). It could also be seen as indicative of a tendency to turn the discussion of the treatment of the Deaf community, in a similar way to many contemporary identity-based social movements, towards a more victim-oriented discourse.

The reaction against hearing aids and cochlear implants is not only due to a fear over the perceived threat to the continued existence of the Deaf community, it is also seen as reinforcing the inferior status of deaf people in the here and now. The proclaiming of such technical advances as 'cures' that will allow the deaf the opportunity to be 'normal' is seen as upholding the abnormal and inferior status of deaf people. As such, it is held to be an attack on the self-worth of deaf people, a direct attack on the integrity of the deaf self. Jankowski notes how many deaf people, if offered some form of medication or treatment that would allow them to hear, would prefer to remain deaf. For them, deafness is a crucial aspect of their self-worth.

In such accounts it is surely a choice for the individuals involved. However, there is an element of narcissism that comes through in such accounts in which such individuals' sense of diminished self-worth can be articulated into an attack on the wishes of not only those who disagree with them, but also on those who would prefer to be able to hear and therefore wish to try whatever technological and/or medical procedures that could provide them with such an opportunity. Despite such problems there is much to commend the Deaf community for the way it presented itself as a campaigning, assertive and political movement that saw the struggle for power as being integral to the concept of empowerment. As we will see later, contemporary articulations are far removed from such radicalism.

When identities collide: intersectionality

One weakness of the focus on identity as a form of political mobilisation is that people are not solely one identity, and neither does any identity comprise a homogenous group of people; the various oppressed identities also overlap. In recognition of this, Kimberlie Crenshaw coined the term 'intersectionality' to illustrate the intersections of various forms of oppression on individual and sub-group experience (Crenshaw, 1989). In the intervening years the term has proven extremely influential amongst many political activists.

The ideas embedded within intersectionality were not new, as Crenshaw herself acknowledged in an interview for *The New Statesman* magazine, noting that each generation, intellectual sphere and political moment had seen

> African American women who have articulated the need to think and talk about race through a lens that looks at gender, or think and talk about feminism through a lens that looks at race. So this is in continuity with that.
>
> (Quoted in Adewunmi, 2014, online)

The principal idea behind intersectionality is that whilst some people experience oppression on account of various aspects of their identity, it is not possible for these to be understood in isolation. The black man is oppressed on account of his race, the black woman on account of both her race and gender. Crenshaw was concerned that there was a tendency to use a single-axis framework with which to account for both racism and sexism. For her, this amounted to the erasure of the experiences of black women by

> limiting inquiry to the experiences of otherwise-privileged members of the group. For example, in race discrimination cases, discrimination tends to be viewed in terms of sex-or class-privileged Blacks; in sex discrimination cases, the focus is on race – and class-privileged women.
>
> (Crenshaw, 1989, p. 57)

By focusing on the most privileged groups within each oppressed category those who are burdened by multiple oppressions are further marginalised. The flaw with those who see multiple oppressions in isolation is that they fail to see the complex way each is interwoven in such a way that the end result is greater than the sum of its parts. For Crenshaw, 'the intersectional experience is greater than the sum of racism and sexism, any analysis that does not take intersectionality into account cannot sufficiently address the particular manner in which Black women are subordinated' (ibid., p. 58).

Such an analysis is not without merit and Crenshaw gives several examples in relation to employment disputes in 1970s USA, but perhaps the most glaring one is in relation to rape in the early twentieth century. She notes that much feminist analysis has highlighted the way that the law and legal institutions have helped establish and maintain the bounds of a normative sexuality by regulating female behaviour. However, Crenshaw points out that whilst early rape laws protected 'chaste' white women from rape, they did not protect black women as they were deemed to be naturally unchaste.

Whilst identity politics has drawn much criticism for potentially reifying and thereby being unable to transcend difference, for Crenshaw (1993) such analyses miss the point. For her, the problem is the opposite in that 'it frequently conflates or ignores intragroup differences' (p. 1242). So, whilst the intersection between racism and sexism is experienced in black women's lifeworld, it tended to be ignored in both feminist and anti-racist practices. She gives several examples of the way race and gender intersect in relation to domestic violence, highlighting the way that the threat of deportation and/or refusal of permanent residence status can lead women of colour to remain with abusive partners in circumstances unlikely to be faced by white Americans.

A similar issue arises at the intersection of race, gender and sexuality. As Audrey Lorde noted:

> Within the lesbian community I am Black, and within the Black community I am a lesbian. Any attack against Black people is a lesbian and gay issue, because I and thousands of other Black women are part of the lesbian community.
>
> (Lorde, 1983, p. 9)

From this perspective any attack against lesbians and gays is also a black issue, because large numbers of lesbians and gay men are also black. In other words, there is no hierarchy of oppression. Such emphasising of the multifaceted aspect of identity highlights the way in which it is not really possible to ignore their intersections. The life-experiences of black heterosexual women will differ from those of black lesbians; for example, the former can marry in virtually all countries, the latter cannot, and may even face prosecution and death on account of their sexuality.

In similar vein, whilst mainstream feminism was critical of the caring role that women were expected to adopt, black feminist accounts situated caring in the context of slavery and racism and its impact on black women (e.g. hooks, 1981). From this perspective, the decision to care is seen as a humanising response to a racist society that devalued black family life. We can also see such issues at other points of intersection. For example, in relation to disability,

Morris (1991) argues that the feminist focus on unpaid care inadvertently assumes that disabled people are a burden on society and actively undermines disabled people's claims for autonomy and independence. Lloyd (2001) also points out that disabled women's experience of sexuality, caring and nurturing does not sit very neatly with the experiences of non-disabled women. For example, for many disabled women their main concern was not that they were defined mainly as sexual objects and nurturers of children but that even these aspects of human life were denied them; they were seen as asexual and incapable of being parents, often being encouraged to undergo sterilisation or having their children removed from them by social services.

The way people perceive images can also be influenced by their particular experience. For example, one public health campaign used pictures of wheelchairs to show people the possible tragic consequences of accidents caused by drink-driving which had such slogans as 'If you think seat belts are confining, think about a wheelchair' and 'Last summer, 1,057 teenagers got so drunk they couldn't stand up. Ever.'

Wang (1992) found that whist it had the desired effect on a non-disabled person – who spoke of her horror should she have an accident and be confined to a wheelchair – confronted with the same images a wheelchair user said, 'What's so bad about using a wheelchair' (p. 1089)? From the latter's perspective, the use of disability to frighten people into adopting 'healthy' lifestyles might be effective 'for people who buy into the whole idea that disability is negative and significantly diminishes one's quality of life. It's devaluing to the rest of us' (ibid.). For disabled people, an unintended consequence of the advertising campaign was the reinforcement of stigma attached to illness and disability.

The linking together of various strands of oppression is seen as not only being essential in order to understand a person's life situation, it is also seen as being necessary to avoid 'horizontal hostility' (hooks, 1981), a situation where one group blames another for their disadvantaged situation. Nevertheless, the desire to link all oppressions is something that can meet with resistance and there have been many instances whereby some groups have not welcomed any intersectional connections with others. For instance, the feminist Betty Friedan, when President of the National Organization of Women (in the USA), did not want the women's movement to be associated with a growing, and often more militant, lesbian grouping for fear that such an association would hamper the potential for the mainstream, heterosexual, feminist movement to influence the political agenda. Friedan called the radical lesbian faction the 'lavender menace'; although she meant it as a term of ridicule the lesbians rather liked the term and so adopted the name.

It could be argued that at the time, in the late 1960s, Friedan did not want attempts to emphasise female rationality undermined by charges that the movement was infiltrated by lesbian 'man-haters'. It is worth remembering that it was not until 1974 that homosexuality was declassified as a mental disorder by the American Psychiatric Association. A similar distancing was evident in some attempts to unite different strands of disability in the 1990s, with many physically disabled activists hostile to attempts to unite with the mental health user movement (Sayce, 2000). The fear was that such an association with the 'mad' would undermine their own attempts to be seen as rational subjects.

The endless etcetera of difference

The obvious problem with both multiple oppressions and intersectionality theories is what has been termed the 'boundless etcetera of difference' whereby an additional identity can always be added to the existing identification (Heartfield, 2002; Butler, 2006). This is inadvertently highlighted by Lorde when she goes on to position herself as 'a Black, lesbian, feminist, socialist, poet, mother of two including one boy and member of an interracial couple' (Lorde, 2015 [1983], online).

In addition, this rather unseemly bidding for most oppressed status can exclude virtually anyone speaking on anything with which they cannot fully identify. For example, because of their specific experiences of both racism and sexism, their intersectionality, Crenshaw believes that it is black women who are best able to challenge all forms of discrimination. It is easy to see where Crenshaw is coming from here, but her argument can be just as easily used against her. How, for instance, can black (heterosexual) women be said to understand the experiences of, or speak for, black lesbians? Can black lesbian women, oppressed on account of the intersectionality of their race, gender and sexuality understand the experiences of, or speak for, the even more intersectionally oppressed disabled black lesbian ... and so we could go on. So, whilst Crenshaw castigates white feminists for ignoring 'how their own race functions to mitigate some aspects of sexism' (1989, p. 67), Crenshaw could similarly be accused by a black disabled woman of ignoring how her own position as an able-bodied black woman similarly ignores the intersection of disability, gender and race.

Indeed Lutz (2002) formulated 14 axes of difference – gender; sexuality; race/skin colour; ethnicity; nation/state, class; culture; ability; age; sedentariness/origin; wealth; North-South; religion; and stage of social development – and even then admitted that the list is in no way complete as additional categories are added or re-defined. The permutations soon become unmanageable; for example, we can, for arguments sake, have three classes (upper, middle, working), three genders (male/female/trans), three sexualities (hetero/homo/bi), myriad ethnicities (White British; Pakistani, Afro-Caribbean; Indian; Irish) further complicated by dual heritage. Even in this basic and numerically limited example we have $3 \times 3 \times 3 \times 5 = 135$ intersectional permutations. As we add further aspects of identity formation the permutations expand exponentially; we can end up with as many intersections as we have people. To further complicate matters, for some, this focus on people is also problematic as it fails to take into account non-human animals within the intersectional matrix (e.g. Cudworth, 2015).

Such theoretical limitations are acknowledged, Butler (2006 [1990]) noting how 'the theories of feminist identity that elaborate predicates of color, sexuality, ethnicity, class and able-bodiness invariably close with an embarrassed "etc." at the end of the list' (p. 196). Similarly, Ehrenreich (2002) refers to the 'infinite regress problem: the tendency of all identity groups to split into ever-smaller sub groups, until there seems to be no hope of any coherent category other than the individual' (p. 267). Indeed, disrupting such categories of subject identification is at the heart of much postmodern and poststructural thought; by showing the historical and cultural variations of such categories it can be shown that they lack any fixed essence. Once again the influence of Foucault is clear to see, with Butler arguing that

> to expose the foundational categories of sex, gender, and desire as effects of a specific formation of power requires a form of critical inquiry that Foucault, reformulating Nietzsche, designates as 'genealogy'. A genealogical critique refuses to search for the origins of gender, the inner truth of female desire, a genuine or authentic sexual identity that repression has kept from view; rather, genealogy investigates the political stakes in designating as an *origin* and *cause* those identity categories that are in fact the *effects* of institutions, practices, discourses with multiple and diffuse points of origin.
>
> (Butler, 2006, p. xxxi, emphasis in original)

The intention of many proponents of intersectionality was to understand and highlight the complexity of the lived experience of oppression. However, in practice, given the absence of any powerful or unifying social movement, intersectional calls can further estrange people from each other and intensify feelings of individuation and vulnerability. This can lead to competition between people and groups over who is the most worthy recipients of state sympathy and protective action. So, whilst writers such as Lorde insist that there is no hierarchy of the oppressed, a position that is increasingly popular amongst many of today's radicals, in practice this is not the case.

In relation to multicultural education policies in the USA, Gorski and Goodman (2011) argue that there is a hierarchy of oppressions with race-related constructs generally receiving more critical considerations than those related to gender, sexual orientation, class, religion, or disability. Indeed, intersectional politics emerged from a prioritising of race and gender over other identity based issues. Similar developments can also be seen in relation to international politics. For example, in Uruguay the National Women's Institute was lobbied by members of the Afro-women's Support Group for the creation of a Department for Afro-descendant women within the Institute. As would be expected, this had a primary focus on the intersections of race and gender. However other activists emphasised the equal or greater importance of other intersections such as sexuality, class, ability and migrant status, whilst others felt the issue of poverty was the defining concern facing the marginalised. Other departments within the Institute emphasised yet other possible intersections such as women with HIV and AIDS, female prisoners, lesbian visibility and lesbophobia alongside the intersection of gender and poverty (Townsend-Bell, 2014). The Australian Human Rights Commission argues that 'an intersectional approach asserts that aspects of identity are indivisible and that speaking about race and gender in isolation from each other results in concrete disadvantage' (AHRC, 2001, online). Within gay politics there seems to be an ever-growing list of letters to describe the movement. Whereas people used to refer to the Lesbian and Gay community, then bisexual was added, followed by transgender, queer and intersex so that many writers now refer to the LGBTQI community or LGBTQI issues.

Attempts to overcome such conceptual difficulties for social and political analyses have tended to adopt a form of 'strategic essentialism' (Spivak, 1996) or critical realism (Bhaskar, 1989) whereby the abandonment of a positivist epistemology does not mean that anything goes. Even in a post-structural landscape it is possible to understand and theorise society in the knowledge that 'changes in the patterns of inequality and in the underlying structural conditions of society are dynamic, complex, and contingent but also amenable to explanation' (McCall, 2009, p. 66).

Despite its theoretical and practical difficulties, the concept of intersectionality has proven extremely influential within many of the new social movements of the latter decades of the twentieth century, many of which came to prominence not from any internal dynamic but rather filled the vacuum left by the decline of the class-based organised labour movement (Heartfield, 2002). However, the new political groupings have had to pay a price for the loss of a class anchor. The early manifestations of identity politics, whilst critical of class analyses that ignored or downplayed issues such as gender or race, still tended to have a strong focus on class, often to the extent of working towards proletarian revolution. Class provided, to a greater or lesser degree, a social anchor, a shared space for society's discontents. As class-based political movements have receded, the common ground on which grievances and strategies could be developed has dissolved. As Bauman (2013) notes, political groupings based on gender, race or other cultural identity, without the anchorage of class have seen a disparate number of grievances aired but they lack the integrative powers of class that had, in theory at least, purported to be a unifying meta-identity. In short, devoid of a universalising anchor there runs the risk, despite the intentions of many of its proponents, of intersectional politics being reconfigured as identity politics which then leads to an internecine battle at the apex of the hierarchy of the oppressed, a process that requires the cultivation of a fragile, inward-looking, vulnerable identity rather than that of a robust political agent with the potential to change the self and society. Unfortunately, such fears have become a feature of much contemporary political activism.

Conclusion: silence as empowerment

The political and theoretical articulation and expression of intersectionality has been defined as an 'analysis-in progress' that rather than being fixed to any particular social position is a theory that develops and moves (Carbado *et al.*, 2013, p. 304). This is a very pertinent point in that it alerts us to the necessity of not focusing on the theory per se but how it is expressed in interaction with the contemporary socio-political environment.

If critical theory is best understood as the theoretical articulation of the political struggles of the day, then we should expect changes in wider society to affect the way intersectionality and claims to empowerment are expressed today. It should be no surprise that traditions forged in one historical era are reconceptualised and reconfigured as they interact with a changing social and political world.

This is something Crenshaw herself acknowledges in conversation with other noted early intersectional theorists Nira Yuval-Davis and Michelle Fine, where she points out that 'a lot of people read intersectionality as just multiplying identity categories rather than constituting a structural analysis or a political critique', and that at times she cannot recognise it in the literature anymore (Guidroz and Berger, 2009, p. 70). In addition, at a macro level the discourse of intersectionality is often used to legitimise Western intervention in other countries, Yuval-Davis pointing out the way that the invasion of Afghanistan and Iraq by the USA and Britain during the 2000s was often legitimised via an intersectional analysis 'about women, Muslim women, and women who need to be rescued by the "enlightened West"' (ibid., p. 77). She goes on to lament the co-option of erstwhile radical discourses around feminism and anti-racism which have been institutionalised and co-opted into legitimising an imperialist and neo-liberal agenda, and how the discourse of 'total inclusiveness' has depoliticised many of the issues initially highlighted by radical political activists.

It has been pointed out that in the present period Politics (with a capital P), is often replaced by politics (with a small p), whereby the focus is on the more micropolitical world at a time when more macro issues are seen as beyond the scope of radical political aspirations (McLaughlin, 2008). Sadly, for many contemporary intersectionalists, this has resulted in their particular standpoint becoming an end in itself, something that is used to bolster rather than transform their particular circumstances. This can be seen in the way that many political interventions do not seek to engage, argue and transform people, ideas and society but, on the contrary, seek to protect and conserve individual identity and ideological beliefs by protecting them from challenge or hurt, often by attempting to stifle debate and silence those with whom they disagree.

Likewise there been an increased sense of individual estrangement and alienation, of what has been termed a 'vulnerability zeitgeist' (Brown, 2015). There has been increased attention to 'microaggressions', which for its advocates constitutes the day-to-day oppression and harassment that they face within society (Wing, 2010). Often this takes the form of a public declaration of hurt to the ego due to being confronted by the more mundane tribulations and misunderstandings that can occur in everyday life. More problematically, rather than confront such incidents, the tendency is often to resort to others – often the police or other regulators – to enforce appropriate civil behaviour, in effect leading to the micromanagement of everyday civil engagement. In an irony that I am sure he would appreciate, and have predicted, Foucault's regulatory regimes are further extended by many of the same people who proclaim they use him to challenge such processes.

One result of all these developments is the desire by many activists today to protect what they see as their own or others' fragile sense of self from the insidious effects of words or actions that can damage their sense of self-worth. It is worth remembering that this was not always the case. In the past, contrary to today, it was not assumed that a subordinated social status automatically rendered someone as feeling worthless, instilling on them low self-esteem. For example, Rollins (1985) observed how the black domestic women she interviewed had kept a strong sense of self-worth despite the psychological attacks on their personhood.

One of the goals of many within radical social movements was the desire to raise the voices of the oppressed. As we saw in Chapters 2 and 3, the power of words was acknowledged and the lack of a voice for many oppressed groups was highlighted. The histories and experiences of the marginalised were to be given a hearing, indeed they were often to be given priority over what was seen as the DWEM dominated literature of politics and academia (DWEM being an acronym for Dead White European Male).

Whilst there was often a censorious aspect to this, with the prioritising of some voices occurring simultaneously with moves to silence others, this was tempered by a desire to raise the numbers of those who could speak and therefore be heard. Today, such voices are increasingly rare and whereas speech was seen as empowering for the oppressed, today it is silence, the power not to hear, that is seen as empowering.

In the UK, veteran activists around such issues as gender and sexuality now find themselves under attack, not by members of the establishment but from a new generation of activists who aim to silence their voices. For example, Julie Bindel, founder of *Women for Justice*, has been prevented from speaking at public debates due to her views on transgender politics. Similarly, Peter Tatchell, founder of *Outrage*, the radical gay campaigning group, has fallen foul of the new censors due to his views not meeting the requirements of the intersectional checklist.

The 'empowerment' of the oppressed is now often seen as best achieved by preventing the utterance of words. University campuses are often where such silencing is most prevalent, where, amongst other things, a wider range of bans have been implemented in order to prevent students from being exposed to ideas, words or images that they may disagree with or find offensive (although, all too often, for many activists, the former is held to be synonymous with the latter). This has led to successful campaigns to prevent speakers with 'controversial' ideas from speaking at universities, seen the banning of popular songs (such as Blurred Lines by Pharrell Williams and Robin Thicke) and newspapers and magazines (such as *The Sun*).

The reason for such censorship is given as the protection of the vulnerable which is more often than not a reference to women, homosexuals, the disabled, ethnic minorities or increasingly those who do not identify with the sex they were born with. This form of empowerment is a far cry from that envisaged by its earlier campaigners. This is not a radical call for the oppressed to challenge dominant ideas by countering them by words and action, but a cry for protection from ideas and words that are seen as harmful to the fragility of both individual and group identity.

What has emerged from the crash at the intersection is not a robust, politically active subject but rather one that is disoriented, shattered and fragile. Whilst it would be a mistake to see this as solely due to the inadequacies of intersectional thinking, the inherent need for identity to be seen in terms of its most vulnerable position, as in the aftermath of a collision, coupled with its ultimately divisive nature, has contributed to the sense of vulnerability and alienation many feel today.

Empowerment as it is conceptualised and framed today has changed significantly in the years since it was first articulated within radical circles. This development can be further illustrated by showing the rise and incorporation of empowerment within the profession of social work. It is this to which we now turn.

4 Empowerment and social work

Introduction

As we have seen, 'empowerment' is a term that is in widespread use today. It has been embraced by the political establishment and proliferates in health, social work and social policy circles. Later, in Chapter 7, we will focus on empowerment as it is understood within health circles, specifically in relation to health promotion. Here I wish to look at the way empowerment began to permeate the related profession of social work. As a 'helping' profession perhaps it should be no surprise to see social work and social workers embrace the concept of empowerment; it could be argued that it is a concept that embodies the values and goals of social work. Indeed, the 'empowerment of users and carers' was one rationale given for the changes to service delivery brought about by the 1990 NHS and Community Care Act (DH/SSI, 1991, p. 7).

However, despite its current ubiquity, the actual term 'empowerment' is a relatively recent addition to contemporary social policy discourse. For example, it was 1986 before it appeared in an original peer-reviewed article in either *Critical Social Policy* (Beuret and Stoker, 1986) or the *British Journal of Social Work* (Ryan, 1986). It would be another three years before another *BJSW* article mentions it (Dominelli, 1989). An archive search of the term I conducted on 26 April, 2012 showed that from its inception in 1971 through to the end of the 1980s, the *BJSW* had only two original articles mentioning empowerment. It was not until 1993 that the term appeared in an abstract (Coulshed, 1993), and 1994 before it appeared in the actual title of an article (Connolly, 1994).

It was the 1990s that saw the idea of empowerment become more and more embedded within social policy and political circles in the UK, to the extent that it is now often used in a rhetorical fashion in such a way that it is held to be a self-evident good, with little elaboration needed on the specific meaning of the term by either the purveyors or recipients of empowerment strategies. The term is now so taken for granted that one book reviewer was critical of the authors for not explicitly referring to it (Lucas, 2006).

Drawing on the work of Smith (2010) and Gomm (1993) I begin with a brief illustration of how power has been articulated in relation to social work. This is meant to supplement the discussion in earlier chapters as well as provide a general overview for those who only read this chapter. There then follows a discussion of empowerment as it has been presented within both social policy and social work circles, noting the roots of the term and some of the factors that have contributed to its widespread adoption. I then take a specific look at the rise and meaning of the term within the *BJSW* from its inception in 1971 until the end of the 1990s. This is due to this being the period that saw empowerment become embedded within UK discourse. My purpose is to provide a chronicle of how wider societal dynamics were being reflected and refracted within what is arguably the UK's most prestigious social work journal concerned with theoretical and practical developments of relevance to the profession.

Power and social work

Within social work there have been many attempts to conceptualise and reframe power relationships. Smith (2010) suggests three formulations of power which he hopes will be of practical help for social workers in addressing the challenges they face: representations of power; modes of power; and sites of power. Within each he further divides them, so representations of power can be distinguished in four ways in which 'power is conceptualised as a material force, but not necessarily as a fixed quantity. It can be viewed as potential; possession; process and product' (online). Power as potential implies the 'capacity to realise change or influence outcomes, which only becomes substantive as it is realised' (ibid.). Power as possession is identified in a more one-sided way with dominant interests, and of how dominant social groups can exercise power in order to secure social order and discipline, but acknowledges that such wielding of power can also be used to offer safeguards and protection to vulnerable individuals or groups. Power as process draws on Bourdieu's (1990) notion of habitus and refers to the fluid nature of power, as something that 'flows between social entities, rather than being held by or located with any one of them', whilst power as product sees power 'not as the instigator or determinant of social relations, but as the outcome of these processes' (Smith, 2010, online).

Modes of power, the means by which power is exercised, are broken down into three; personal, positional and relational. Personal power draws on Weber's notion of charisma, with the rider that personal identity is closely linked to wider power dynamics that can forge and mould identity – for example, around class, gender or ethnic lines. Positional power is connected to the location of power – for example, around professional power – or power invested in an individual by virtue of his or her title. Relational power places an emphasis on an interactive dimension to power relations, something of increasing importance given the competing claims to power, authority and truth in a postmodern world in which traditional sources of authority are frequently challenged. The various sites of power – such as courtrooms, community, social work offices and the home (as social workers' power can extend into the private realm of its clientele) – are also highlighted in order for us to 'recognise that power relations are not uniform or all-pervasive, and their content and forms of enactment will vary according to the setting' (ibid.).

In a similar vein, Gomm (1993) discusses four possible views on power in relation to health, welfare and education services. It can entail an oppressive or a liberating relationship; the former view would argue that health, welfare and education services enable the rich to continue to exploit the poor, maintaining them at a minimum level of efficiency and, echoing the 'false consciousness' instilled by the workings of ideology discussed in Chapter 2, misleading them about the true nature of their societal position. The situation for the workers involved in such services is, in some respects, worse, as

> they are oppressed oppressors. Those who do not recognize this are just as duped by the system as are the users of services. For those who do recognize this, the only proper course of action is to ally themselves with users and challenge the system: to become liberators rather than oppressors.
>
> (p. 133)

In the 'helping relationship' view there is an 'expertise gap' between workers and users, with the former using their expertise in the interests of the user. The third view focuses on ways in which the professional relationship can be disabling rather than enabling – for example, in the way that professionals deny users the facilities and knowledge to do things by themselves. Fourth, is a 'brokerage relationship' which, as the name implies, sees workers as brokers between users and services and other competing community stakeholders.

Even with such a brief consideration of power it will be clear to see how the notion of empowerment would have particular relevance within social work circles and, as will be shown below, social work did indeed embrace empowerment, although there were some dissenting voices.

The rise and meaning(s) of empowerment

As mentioned above, from its inception in 1971 through to the end of the 1980s, the *BJSW* had only two original articles mentioning empowerment. However, there were a couple of references to the term in book reviews prior to 1986, in relation to black and community empowerment respectively. Indeed, one of the earliest attempts at defining empowerment was in relation to social work with Black communities in the USA, where Solomon (1976) defined it as 'a process whereby persons who belong to a stigmatized social category throughout their lives can be assisted to develop and increase skills in the exercise of interpersonal influence and performance of valued social roles' (p. 6). Later definitions broadened the recipients of the empowerment process. So, for Wallerstein (1992) it is

> a social-action process that promotes participation of people, organisations and communities towards the goal of increased individual and community control, political efficacy, improved quality of community life and social justice.
>
> (p. 198, quoted in Anderson, 1996, p. 70)

Such a wide-ranging definition, divorced from the requirement 'to belong to a stigmatized social category', may be useful but it can also allow people to interpret empowerment in any way they choose, in the process making it more difficult to know with clarity what is being done or attempted in its name. Indeed, in an edited book titled *Pathways to Empowerment*, the editor notes in her introduction that it is not possible to give a definitive definition of empowerment as it is a term that is still evolving and also one that means different things to different people, therefore all the book's contributors were free to work to their own definition (Parsloe 1996a). However, despite these slight differences in interpretation, for Parsloe, at its core, empowerment 'involves an increase in the power of users of social services' (ibid., p. xvii).

Clarity of definition has not been achieved in the intervening years. As Adams (2008) notes, empowerment is 'a multifaceted idea, meaning different things to different people' and therefore 'no final, so called "authoritative" definition' is possible (p. 4). Nevertheless, drawing on definitions taken from Thomas and Pierson (1995), Adams (2008) argues that it can be seen as

> the capacity of individuals, groups and/or communities to take control of their circumstances, exercise power and achieve their own goals, and the processes by which, individually and collectively, they are able to help themselves and others to maximize the quality of their lives.
>
> (p. 17)

In practical terms, though, it invariably means authority figures – for example, professionals such as social workers – intervening in order to 'empower' people. In this respect Parsloe (1996b) argued that the term could be seen as not a very appropriate word for social work to have adopted, due to 'the very idea that one person, a social worker, can empower another, a client, runs counter to the whole idea of greater equality of power on which the concept supposedly depends' (p. 6). However, she is also of the belief that it is a process that, in theory at least, involves an increase in the power of those who use social services. This is similar to Thompson's (2007) frustration at those who see power as akin to a zero-sum game when the situation is more nuanced than that; power need not be something someone (a social worker) gives to a client, power can be generative, which means professionals can use their power to generate service user power. For Thompson, the basis of empowering practice is therefore to use professional power 'not to coerce or to suppress, but rather to help people move towards taking greater control over their lives' (p. 24).

In this respect 'empowerment' can be seen as a relatively benign term, a way of helping people gain increased power to organise their affairs and achieve their goals and desires. Nevertheless, a term that has become so embedded within both policy and practice initiatives has also attracted much criticism over what it represents in both theoretical terms and practical social work interactions.

Questioning empowerment

The rise to prominence of the rhetoric of empowerment did not go unnoticed or uncontested. Indeed, the term had its critics even as it was first becoming established. By the early 1990s, some had noticed how the term had become something of a buzz-word that littered the mission statements of health, welfare and education services (Gomm, 1993). Humphries (1996) noted how its mention, directly or by implication, had become 'de rigueur in articles, books and political statements' and that it had 'become a key objective in the training of professionals of all kinds, particularly the caring professions' (p. 1). Such a situation led Humphries to ask, and attempt to answer, the question of why the discourse of empowerment had become so dominant at this historical moment. She highlights the political struggles of the 1980s and the rise and fall of bureaucratic and proceduralist strategies to combat inequality. Such developments differed from the more radical perspectives in that the latter were more concerned with empowerment as being something that emerged through individual and collective action, the former involving a more top-down approach to the alleviation of individual and societal problems.

The wider political context and the way that empowerment can mean different things to different people can be illustrated in relation to sexuality and gender. For some it manifested as demands for women to gain control over their own bodies in relation to such things as sexual self-definition and control over their own fertility, for others, more emphasis was placed on sexual pleasure and freedom, whilst for lesbian and gay activists empowerment meant the right to be visible and to be treated equally in society (Carabine, 1996). Nevertheless, one key shared aim was on women (and lesbians and gay men) empowering themselves (Ramazanoglu and Holland, 1993).

In a similar vein, Langan (1998) pointed out that during the 1970s radical activists had a commitment to the 'self-activity' of the working class. In such a climate of collective working class action the notion of philanthropy implied by the bestowal of power by professionals on the working class was not particularly resonant; the belief was that members of the working class were capable of organising themselves, of gaining power from below by virtue of their collective strength, not having it sprinkled onto them from above like confetti. In this respect,

> the rise of the concept of empowerment and its institutionalisation within social work theory and practice is reflective of both the decline of working class collective power and the changing conception of 'empowerment'; from something to be taken, by force if necessary, to something to be handed down by the state, here in the guise of the social worker.
>
> (McLaughlin, 2015, p. 97)

This did not preclude people aligning themselves with oppressed and disadvantaged groups. It was not about non-engagement but about joining together to achieve mutually desirable goals, perhaps best summed up by the following quote attributed to an Aborigine women: 'If you are here to help me then you are wasting your time. But if your liberation is tied up with mine, then let us begin' (quoted in Anderson, 1996, p. 69).

Such suspicion of 'benevolent' help is justified, as far from being a benign term empowerment can actually be a vehicle for far from progressive social policies and practical implementation. For Rees, 'the word "empowerment" has been and is being used as a term of convenience, to justify the maintenance of disempowering policies and practices rather than to their elimination' (quoted in Wai Man, 1996, p. 45). In addition, this relatively new concept 'is being substituted for old ones without the political nature of empowerment being developed' (ibid.). In other words, at a time when previous political movements around such things as race and gender were receding there was more of a focus on the individual whereby 'empowerment' became the goal, but one that lacked substance or political analysis. In this sense it represents a depoliticising of action for change, a wider political outlook being replaced with a more individualistic casework notion of empowerment.

For Ward and Mullender (1993) empowerment needs to be connected with a notion of oppression in order to become a distinctive underpinning for practice. This is because, for them, whilst empowerment often means little more than 'enabling', oppression 'can be understood both as a state of affairs in which life chances are constructed, and as a process by which this state of affairs is created and maintained' (p. 148).

It is difficult to think that in the 1980s anti-racism and multiculturalism were distinct terms, with the former being more concerned with issues of power than culture, with the macropolitical and economic rather than the more micro personal issues. Indeed, anti-racism and multiculturalism were often in conflict In relation to social work education. Naik (1993) note how 'anti-racist education is interested in power, rather than culture, the political and economic, rather than mere social work issues and in changing the social and educational structures, rather than the social worker's sensitivities' (p. 84).

The contemporary notion of empowerment as a process that allows service users to have more control over their lives can also prove illusory. In reality it can be a mechanism for drawing people into participating in processes and decisions over which they have little meaningful control. As Langan (1998) notes,

> Parents are said to be empowered by being invited to attend child protection case conferences; they thus become complicit in measures of state intervention in their family life decided on by professionals and the police. Applicants for community care are empowered by the fact that their designated social worker is also the manager of a devolved budget which is limited by criteria quite independent of the applicant's needs. Too often, empowerment means reconciling people to being powerless.

(p. 215)

To this we could add the way in which psychiatric patients are 'empowered' by being encouraged to contribute to their care plan, but with the introduction of the Mental Health Act 2007 their power to refuse prescribed medication post-discharge is often not up for discussion. In other words, the power that is given (arguably a contradiction in terms) is bound within certain parameters, and these can lead to a lowering of expectations as well as being predicated on the client ultimately being submissive to those who, in reality, wield power.

If the empowerment process can undermine individual autonomy there are also those who are wary of its relationship to a form of individualism which they associate with political conservatism and self-help, as opposed to equality and liberatory based group politics around such things as anti-racism, feminism and class. However, as Adams (2008) points out, the more radical approaches also emphasised self-help – for example, radical psychiatric patients/activists emphasised action to free themselves and not to rely on therapists or social workers.

The notion of empowerment entails a relationship between someone who is held to be relatively powerless in a given context compared to another person who is seen to be able to help them to gain some degree of power over whatever aspect of their live is presented as a problem. In this sense it is not something done to the person, rather they are said to be enabled to empower themselves (Thompson, 2007). However, as we have seen, empowerment can involve both liberatory and regulatory measures as it becomes incorporated into professional discourse and can be used to justify professionals' positions and their preferred method of intervention (Baistow, 1995).

The discussion above has briefly highlighted the rise, justifications for and criticisms of the concept of empowerment. In what follows I wish to illustrate how the term was discussed within the pages of the *BJSW* during the 1980s and 1990s, specifically in original peer-reviewed articles as opposed to book reviews or critical commentaries that discuss work published external to the journal. My interest is in describing and highlighting the way in which external developments began to permeate social work discourse and, in turn, how social work moulded them for its own purposes.

Empowerment and the *British Journal of Social Work*

Given the development of empowerment as a concept and political strategy in wider society it will be instructive to detail how this was reflected within social work. The *British Journal of Social Work* is arguably the UK's most prestigious social work journal. As such, it is revealing to look at the way the term empowerment emerged and developed within the pages of the journal. In so doing I will describe the way it grew in popularity and also identify the different conceptual models that were used in the development and articulation of the term. However, as we shall see, the majority of the analysis has to focus on the 1990s due to empowerment not being in popular usage during the first two decades of the *BJSW*'s existence.

The *BJSW* was first published in 1971. However, it was not until the ninth edition in 1979, in a review of the book *Black Empowerment: Social Work in Oppressed Communities* by Barbara Bryant Solomon that the word 'empowerment' appears for the first time anywhere within its pages. This book's predominant focus was on developments in the USA (Cheetham, 1979). In 1985, in another book review 'community empowerment' is mentioned as a possible strategy in working with people, again illustrated by examples from the USA (Service, 1985).

It was in a supplementary edition of the 1986 volume that the first original article appeared that specifically mentioned empowerment. The article looked at interventions with young mothers who were experiencing depression, and recognised the role of wider support networks in its alleviation. Such 'community empowerment' was seen as a strategy 'to decrease the sense of apathy and helplessness of the user group by maximizing the probability that initiatives taken by the families, however small, met with successful outcomes', and implied 'giving families a real say in how resources are both allocated and spent' (Ryan, 1986, p. 79).

A 1987 book review, again concerned with the USA, notes the authors' mention of 'political empowerment' as being a wholly client-centred approach (Rossetti, 1987), whilst the following year, another book review notes that the issue of 'community empowerment' is not one that has been much pursued in the UK (Cooper, 1988).

The first and only detailed discussion of the concept of empowerment during the first two decades of the *BJSW*'s existence appears in 1989 in an article on incest abuse and power relationships from a feminist perspective (Dominelli, 1989). Feminist empowerment in this context is said to consist of four major thrusts. The first is concerned with providing women and children with individual support. The second concentrates on enabling abused girls and women to come together in groups. The third thrust attempts to get groups of abused women to acknowledge the social divisions which exist between them, whilst the fourth thrust challenges the punitive treatment incest victims/survivors are said to be subjected to once investigations for criminal proceedings against their assailants are initiated.

Nevertheless, despite Dominelli's intervention, it is clear that empowerment was a rarely discussed concept within the *BJSW* during this period. However, this was to change markedly during the following decade.

The 1990s: empowerment goes mainstream

As noted above, the 1990s saw empowerment come of age in wider social and political discourse, and although this is reflected to an extent in the *BJSW* detailed discussion was mainly to be found in books and other print formats. For example, whilst 1990 saw the term mentioned in two articles (Fielden, 1990; Braye and Preston-Shoot, 1990) there was no definition given or discussion around it. The following year, in an article concerned with the professionalisation of social work and the setting up of a general council, Hugman (1991) sees a stark choice for social workers 'between the opportunity for empowering the profession in its current path of professionalisation on the one hand and using social work for the joint empowerment of professionals and service users on the other' (p. 213). Hugman would prefer to see collective service user representation on any such professional organisation.

The early 1990s also saw empowerment being discussed in relation to more distinct groups. It is said to be about 'consumer choice' (Hatfield *et al.*, 1992) and an essential component of both challenging and extending the normalisation process in relation to community care and user and carer participation (Smith and Brown, 1992; Hughes, 1993). The need for 'student empowerment' is also highlighted (e.g. de Maria, 1992) with the values of empowerment said to underpin self-directed learning (Taylor, 1993). According to Coulshed (1993) it was a requirement of the then new Diploma in Social Work that social work education fosters empowerment. There is even an acknowledged need for 'a new doctrine of empowerment' (Smith and Brown, 1992, p. 686), although as we reach the end of 1992 we have still not had any substantial discussion in the *BJSW* of what the old doctrine was.

The following year saw the first article to have the word empowerment in the title (Connolly, 1994). The article is about 'family decision making' legislation and practice in New Zealand. However, whilst it appears in the title, the only other reference to it is contained in the summary/introduction which claims that the process aims to tackle family disempowerment. Empowerment then is an attempt to address disempowerment, but still there is no specific discussion or clarification as to what such terms actually mean.

For Boushell (1994) the focus on empowerment was very fragmented in nature despite 'recent theoretical developments in antidiscrimination and user empowerment' (p. 188). This is the only time the word appears in the article; however, its positioning further informs us that the issue of empowerment was 'out there', being discussed in social, political and academic circles. This is partially addressed later in 1994 when there is more of an attempt to offer a definition or explanation of what empowerment entails, even if, as in the following two citations the actual word empowerment only appears once in each article. Howe (1994) sees the growth of a concern with participation and empowerment as taking place within a wider framework of postmodern scepticism towards truth and a neo-conservative focus on freedom and the individual, whilst for Cnaan (1994) 'empowerment is more than the legal right to perform certain functions; it is a process that educates and helps clients to make independent decisions and care for themselves' (p. 542).

Whilst we are now beginning to get more elaboration on what empowerment actually means, nevertheless it is still the case that into the 1990s no article contributors to the *BJSW* have felt the need to give a detailed explanation of the term or indeed competing or critical explanations. What comes through within these early discussions of empowerment is that, contrary to Thompson's (2007) fears discussed above, it is apparent that power is not necessarily viewed as a zero-sum game; on the contrary the articles, either explicitly or implicitly, view it as being potentially a generative process, whereby strategies of empowerment can lead to increased power for all involved. Service users gaining power does not necessarily detract from social workers' power, both can potentially benefit from a more representational and dialogic arrangement.

The value of education and Habermasian communicative ideals is evident within much of the discussions over how best to achieve this holy grail of 'empowerment'. However, some concern was raised – for example, Corby *et al.* (1996) note that 'the emphasis on partnership and empowerment raises false expectations in many parents' raising many ethical considerations and that far from 'achieving the goal of engaging parents and helping them to care better for their children, it could alienate them and make them apathetic' (p. 489).

It was in the second half of the 1990s that the concept of empowerment began to be more widely mentioned and critically evaluated. Its growing popularity not only in Western Europe but in Eastern Europe was also noted (Ramon, 1995). This is further evidence that the theme of empowerment was gaining in relevance both within and outside the academy, and that social work is not only greatly influenced by wider social and political developments but does, albeit to a lesser degree, adapt and reflect back to society aspects of these modifications.

Critical approaches to empowerment

For Calder (1995), empowerment had become a trendy notion that can operate as a form of social control and that therefore its image of equality and openness is misleading, since the distribution of power is clearly unequal. Meanwhile, within social work education the move towards a competency model of social work was seen as potentially leading to 'forms of intervention which further disempower users whilst clothing their activities in the rhetoric of citizenship and empowerment' (Dominelli, 1996, p. 173). For Humphries (1997), its 'seductiveness is in the *co-option* of liberal humanist discourse of "student-centred learning", but this is tied into centrally determined, predefined goals' (p. 650, emphasis in original). In addition, influenced by the intersectional perspective we discussed in the previous chapter, it was argued that the focus of 'empowerment' in relation to only one aspect of a person's life – for example, impairment, age or psychiatric diagnosis – can miss other issues such as race, class and gender that can contribute to the person's lack of power.

This co-option can be seen in relation to mental health services. As Forbes and Sashidharan (1997) note, many hospital mental health advocacy groups not only contributed unrewarded user energy and labour they also did little to change the environment or provide alternatives for those who found the existing service set-up unhelpful. Many psychiatric user-run services had compromised so much in exchange for funding and 'a seat at the table' that they could be hard to distinguish from mainstream mental health services. Similarly, Browne (1996) sees empowerment as about giving a voice to survivors of child abuse and treating survivor organisations as equal contributors to resolving issues arising from the abuse, but cautions that they can have their views subordinated to those of professionals due to the current hierarchical set up of services.

Bland (1997) is the first *BJSW* contributor to give the concept of empowerment some detailed discussion. Drawing on the work of Adams (1990), she notes that dictionary definitions of the verb 'to empower' are wide-ranging and include 'to invest legally or formally with power', to 'authorize or license', 'to impart power to do something', and 'to enable or permit'. She agrees with Adams' view that the last definition is the least radical and that it is probably the one which is most often implied in social work, noting that to

> 'impart power' to someone implies an actor with power giving up some of that power to another, with freedom to use it as they wish. To 'enable or permit' implies a more restricted relinquishing of power within a framework approved by the donor.
>
> (Bland, 1997, p. 588)

For Bland, residents' rights and charters are forms of positive empowerment that have been developed for older people in residential care. Whilst Bland's approach can be read as endorsing a weak version of the zero-sum concept of power it is arguably one that is close to the reality of social work practice.

Empowerment as resource substitute

According to Lewis *et al.* (1997), empowerment is one of a variety of 'instruments for facilitating person-centred resource allocation and decision-making' (p. 3), although they do note the conflict of interest between user-empowerment and resource allocation. In such circumstances people can be 'empowered' into accepting poor or inadequate service provision as they are drawn into mechanisms of resource prioritisation and allocation. This more sceptical view is echoed by Clark (1998), who views empowerment as a fashionable concept that has become excessively elastic and that has had little useful impact. The use, and potential misuse, of Western notions of empowerment for Africa and African people is also discussed with the dangers of ethnocentrism and missionary zeal being highlighted (Bar-On, 1999; Graham, 1999).

The potential, contradictions and dangers of the way empowerment is conceptualised and implemented began to be articulated and developed as the 1990s developed. Arguably the most detailed discussion of empowerment is by Lupton (1998) in an article about Family Group Conferences. She notes how the concept contains

> both a rights-based and a responsibility-based interpretation of the relationship between the individual and the state. It may not only involve individuals striving for greater power and control over their lives, but may also require those individuals to develop a greater degree of independence and self-reliance.
>
> (Lupton, 1998, p. 110)

For her, such objectives are not necessarily contradictory, it being possible that enabling individuals to meet their own needs can enhance their sense of gaining control over their circumstances, of feeling empowered, although she warns of the possible tension if the promotion of self-reliance is primarily concerned with reducing expenditure on state provided services. Rather than embrace or reject empowerment per se, '[i]deas or initiatives that claim empowerment as a central objective therefore require careful scrutiny to assess the particular combination of rights and responsibilities by which they are underpinned' (ibid.).

Conclusion

This chapter has charted the growing popularity of the concept of empowerment within social policy and social work, with a more specific detailing of its rise in the *British Journal of Social Work* from 1971–1999. The chosen timeframe allowed us to see the development of empowerment through the pages and history of the journal during the period from the journal's inception to the end of the decade in which empowerment became firmly embedded in social, political and professional discourse. As such it is more of a historically descriptive account rather than a deep theoretical analysis. However, it should be clear that the discourse of empowerment did not come from nowhere, but rather was influenced by wider social and political change. The meaning of empowerment, whilst never fixed, indeed often used but rarely defined, was subject to change and contestation. Detailing these issues is important if we are to understand the origins of contemporary discursive practices.

It is tempting to think of empowerment as just being a nice contemporary term for activities that have always formed the basis of good social work. As Jackson (1996) puts it, in reference to social work practice in the 1960s, 'Though, thirty years on, we may call it empowerment, it is still the combination of practical help and the quality of the relationship that enables social workers, sometimes, to help people change their lives for the better' (p. 50). Similarly, Parsloe (1996b) argues that whilst professionals may not give a detailed analysis of what empowerment is, in practice they tend to share the desire 'to assist or encourage clients to develop the confidence, competence and self-esteem' to have a greater say in the provision, planning and creation of the services they want (p. 8).

Nevertheless, there is a danger that such a term can be utilised so often that its meaning and application in a given context is taken as an a priori good. As has been shown in relation to strategies around 'anti-oppression', feel good rhetoric can be used to hide behind far from progressive policies and practice (Humphries, 2004). In this respect it is important to not only historicise empowerment, to show its conditions of emergence, but also to look at what is being done in its name in the here and now.

5 From consciousness-raising to awareness-raising

Introduction

In this chapter I wish to revisit the concept of ideology and consciousness we discussed in Chapters 2 and 3 in relation to postmodern conceptions of power and the strategies adopted by the more radical early campaigners in their drive towards empowerment. The issue of ideology and the workings of power that it can disguise were highlighted and in the process the boundaries of what constituted such areas as the political, public and private spheres were called into question.

The problem for many political activists was how to remove the ideological blinds from the oppressed and enable them to see the true nature of their oppression, to allow them to see the shadows on Plato's cave for what they truly are – shadows, a reflection of reality and not reality itself. The consciousness-raising activities that emerged often sought to develop a shared, collective understanding of 'personal' and political issues, from which a theoretical framework through which to view societal relationships would emerge. However, such ostensibly organic initiatives were also vulnerable to the proclamations of those who saw themselves as the bearers of 'true' consciousness, who saw their role as being to educate the masses out of their 'false' consciousness.

As will be clear by now, a key theme of this book is the importance of understanding the changing nature of political articulation and struggle over the past 50 years. This chapter further develops this by showing how, latterly, 'consciousness-raising' as it was previously understood has become increasingly rare in relation to political discourse. Today, with the demise of the radical movements that championed the need to awaken the masses from their slumber, the public, political and civic spheres have become dominated by campaigners who are more likely to talk about their role being about raising the awareness of the population. This awareness-raising is rarely connected to wider socio-political issues and tends to be preoccupied with interpersonal issues or health and behaviour oriented forms of intervention.

As I will show below, and in subsequent chapters, the move from consciousness-raising to awareness-raising is not simply a matter of semiotics but reflects the changing nature of political struggle and ideological articulation in the contemporary period.

Ideology and consciousness

In its contemporary left-wing usage empowerment emerged alongside the radical political movements of the 1960s particularly in the USA. These 'new social movements' challenged the idea of a unique space of the political by questioning the narrow terrain of constitutional politics and problematizing the notion of any clear distinction between the political, social and personal. The 'political' was moved from a narrow focus on overt conflict to those terrains where it is uncontested due to the working of power and ideology. A lack of overt political resistance to issues such as poverty and inequality is not seen as indicating the depoliticisation of such issues. On the contrary, 'to say that welfare and bureaucratic modes of government "depoliticize" the political exclusion of welfare recipients is to mistake the absence of resistance for an absence of politics' (Cruikshank, 1999, p. 5). Echoing Judith Butler, Cruikshank emphasises that the subject, even one who does not resist, is herself a political subject, and as such is 'perhaps most political at the point in which it is claimed to be prior to politics itself' (ibid., p. 5). From such a perspective it is not a case of focusing on the micro at the expense of the macro political but of intervening in the pre-political as that is where the workings of power are most insidious.

This acknowledgement that any system of oppression derives much of its strength from the acquiescence of its victims, who have internalised and accepted the dominant image of themselves and are thus paralysed by a sense of helplessness, led many radicals to look at ways in which the true nature of oppression could be revealed. Liberation strategies, therefore, are concerned with helping the oppressed to see the reality of their oppression, of helping them see that problems such as ill health, homelessness, unemployment or poverty are not due to individual weakness or pathology but to do with the way in which society is organised in the interests of the powerful. A process of consciousness-raising is called for to help the oppressed see behind the ideological facade of prevailing social relations. Of course, this assumes a belief on behalf of the consciousness-raisers that they hold true knowledge and that they have a duty to pass this knowledge to the unenlightened (as we will see in later chapters, such sentiments can soon morph into a disdain for those who fail to adopt the 'correct' form of consciousness).

As we discussed in Chapter 3, empowerment, in its early manifestation, was inherently connected to campaigns, discussions and strategies aimed at raising the consciousness of individuals or groups of people, often from oppressed or marginalised groups, in pursuit of a wider political project to change some or other aspect of society. The work of writers such as Paulo Friere, particularly his 1970 book, *The Pedagogy of the Oppressed*, proved highly influential, especially on left-leaning academics, because of its analysis of the role of education in the maintenance of oppressive social relationships and the need for a critical awareness to develop amongst the poor and disadvantaged. Women's groups set up 'consciousness-raising' groups whereby women would share personal experiences which would allow the political aspects of such experiences to be exposed in a process that would see the development of a collective consciousness that made sense of what were hitherto felt to be individual problems.

The Women's Liberation Movement used personal examples to draw conclusions about the political nature of such 'personal' issues. It was a tactic/process that was used extensively in the 1970s and was seen as a crucial element in developing a critical awareness of the inter-relationship between the personal/political and public/private spheres. One key theorist of what became known as 'feminist standpoint theory' was Nancy Hartsock who attempted to reconcile feminism and Marxism by rearticulating historical materialism via the prism of women's experiences. For her, the aim of feminist epistemology was to develop knowledge from experience. In this reading, theory is 'appropriated experience' (Hartsock, 1998, p. 38) and consciousness-raising highlighted and connected 'personal experience to the structures that define our lives' (ibid., p. 35). Such initiatives entailed a direct critique of the prevailing social system, but this more radical agenda failed to achieve wider resonance with the majority of women, as hooks (1984) acknowledges:

> Feminist consciousness-raising has not significantly pushed women in the direction of revolutionary politics. For the most part, it has not helped women understand capitalism – how it works as a system that exploits female labor and its interconnections with sexist oppression. It has not urged women to learn about different political systems like socialism or encouraged women to invent and envision new political systems.... Most importantly, it has not continually confronted women with the understanding that feminist movement to end sexist oppression can be successful only if we are committed to revolution, to the establishment of a new social order.
>
> (p. 161)

In similar vein, Sowards and Renegar's (2004) analysis of the changing rhetorical strategies of second and third wave feminists notes how the latter 'offer their stories and experiences, but do not necessarily expect a social movement to develop as a result' (p. 548). As I have argued elsewhere, due to the loss of faith in the ability to achieve wider social change activists increasingly focused their attentions on the more micro aspects of life but in the process the personal is political slogan, whilst still used rhetorically, in practice got reversed so that the political became increasingly restricted to the personal sphere, with consciousness-raising being transformed into a more therapeutic analysis of the self (McLaughlin, 2012). As we see in Chapter 7, this form of personal change also began to take on a more health-oriented focus; after all, health is something we can all relate to as a personal issue.

In her analysis of the development of empowerment, Cruikshank (1999) argues that what we have seen is a reconceptualization of the 'social'. For her, the social sphere

> is not the space traversed between citizens and the state; it is neither the space of uncoerced association (as in 'civil society') nor the space of

conformity and domination (as in "social control"). Rather, the social confuses and reconstitutes the boundaries between the personal and the political, the economy and the state, the voluntary and the coercive.

(p. 6)

This breaking down of boundaries, with the social being seen as an object of reform, measurement and intervention can be seen as dislocating the political from its spatial association with the sovereign and the state. However, new and arguably more powerful forms of power emerge.

Cruikshank notes that the political logic of empowerment can dichotomise power and powerlessness, with people being labelled one or the other. Her focus is not on empowerment per se but on relations of empowerment, which for her include four characteristics. First, empowerment entails a relationship based on expertise, albeit that such expertise is frequently contested (e.g. the expertise of professionals conflicting with the lived expertise of their clients, something that can be seen within the radical mental health movement). Second, it is a democratically unaccountable exercise of power due to the relationship often being initiated by one party, usually professionals or activists, seeking to empower another. Third, it uses social scientific models to gather 'knowledge' of those to be empowered. Fourth, the process of empowerment is simultaneously both voluntary and coercive. In addition, the 'self-help' referred to by promoters of empowerment does not refer to autonomous selves helping others but that the government intervenes to create relations of help between these otherwise disparate selves.

Dean (1999) highlights what he sees as the advantage of Cruikshank's analysis compared to that of Fraser and Gordon's (1994) genealogy of the discourse surrounding welfare dependency. Fraser and Gordon adopt a form of analysis known as 'ideological critique', whereby they seek to reveal the ideological underpinnings of language. Informed by the Frankfurt School of Critical Theory, the aim is to reveal the possibility of alternative emancipatory ways of thinking. For Dean (1999), such an approach is problematic as it regards language as a 'second-order phenomenon shaped by more fundamental forces and conditions' (p. 64). Such an overly structural approach underestimates the role of language in the construction of social worlds and individual subjectivity. 'Key terms in the vocabularies of rule – such as dependency – are not simply ideological condensations of the meanings of broad social structures. They are integral components of government, of our organized systems of acting upon and directing human conduct' (ibid.).

In displacing the centrality of ideology critique, Dean argues that there is a need for forms of analysis that move on from categories such as 'sole parent' and 'long-term unemployed', that are contingent on changing social structures, to a focus on how such categories arise from, and are integral to, particular regimes of practice in relation to the provision of welfare. He also argues that we need to disabuse ourselves of the notion that a demystification of such welfare terms will allow us to uncover real relations of subordination. Whilst such an argument runs the risk of underestimating the structural power of government, Dean's third point is a very pertinent one where he argues that 'we should reject the romanticization of the "victim" often coupled with the critique of ideology' (Dean, 1999, p. 66).

A key criticism of Fraser and Gordon's position is that they fail to see how the art of government often relies on the very agency of the governed themselves, which can blind them to the danger that ostensibly emancipatory practices or sites of resistance can themselves be co-opted into the disciplinary process. To illustrate this further, Dean (1999) compares Fraser and Gordon's position with that of Cruikshank (1994) who uses Foucauldian theory to analyse the Community Action Programs (CAP) in 1960s USA. CAPs emerged as part of the 'War on Poverty' initiative of President Johnson and the aim was to help communities to help themselves, or in contemporary discourse, the goal was empowerment. This entailed what Cruikshank refers to as a technology of citizenship that entails the transformation of the subjectivity of the poor from one of powerlessness and inertia to that of active citizenship. The idea that it is necessary to empower 'victims' in order that they will engage in a more active way with welfare agencies, and in the process overcome a passive, dependent relation to government, was not only a bulwark of government policy discourse it was also a key component of the emerging New Left activism of the time.

One outcome of the US 'War on Poverty' was that the issue of poverty became redefined from something resulting not from the actions of the powerful but from the inaction of the poor, a viewpoint that united both those in government and the more radical community activists. As she summarises,

> The 'apathy' of the poor was for the New Left, as it was for liberal reformers, the central and continuing cause of their poverty and unequal status. The key to revolution and reform alike was understood to be in the independent and voluntary participation of the poor in their own emancipation.
>
> (Cruikshank, 1999, p. 76)

Cruikshank's analysis is insightful but in the contemporary period it is not the case that radicals, reformers and conservatives uphold the belief in 'the independent and voluntary participation of the poor'. As we will see in the following chapters, all political hues tend to coalesce around the belief that 'the poor', indeed all social demographics, require guidance and/or censure in order to achieve not emancipation, but an ill-defined 'healthy citizenship'. Today, whilst the need for such 'consciousness-raising' can occasionally be heard, it has, for the most part, been marginalised within social and political campaign discourse. Today, you are far more likely to encounter an individual or group trying to raise your awareness, not your consciousness.

The transition from 'consciousness-raising' to 'awareness-raising' is no mere change in vocabulary with little wider social, cultural or political meaning. On the contrary, the ascendancy of 'awareness-raising' is related to the changing sociocultural context of contemporary society. Often, those in the business of awareness raising – and as we shall see, 'business' is an apposite description – whilst often influenced by, and concerned with, the issues taken up by the old and new social movements of yesteryear, cannot be termed social movements in the traditional sense as they lack any real connection with the public they seek to empower. In addition, there are negative implications for social policy from the rise of such groups and the way they seek to promote their particular cause, often exaggerating the extent of their particular issue in order to get their cause more publicity and funding.

The rise of awareness raising

The rise of awareness-raising campaigns can be seen in the way that there is barely a day in the year that is not allocated a specific cause to highlight, with some commanding an even longer period in the awareness calendar. The whole of January 2014 was 'Love Your Liver' month, part of the 'Love your Liver' campaign, a national awareness initiative run by the British Liver Trust. March 2014 saw 'World Orphan Week' which hoped to raise awareness of the issues facing orphans in poorer countries. A cursory glance at Project Britain's calendar of awareness events shows us that in March 2015 alone we have numerous awareness raising events including 'Brain Awareness Week', 'World Glaucoma Week' and 'World Kidney Day'. There appears to be a hierarchy of organs evident here, the liver getting a month, the brain a week and the poor kidney getting just a solitary day. As the year goes on we will have our awareness raised about many other things such as child abuse, alcohol misuse, stress and a variety of mental health problems. We also are informed of many subgroups within these categories so, for example, not only do we have cancer awareness but we also have its offshoots, with, for example the 15–21 September, 2014 being designated 'Lymphatic Cancer Awareness Week'. According to the charity behind this campaign there was a problem in that many people were unaware of lymphoma until they or a loved one developed the disease.

Often, awareness campaigns are presented as a form of political action; by raising people's awareness of a particular issue campaigners maintain that they are empowering people to take control over their lives. So, according to Laura Bates, founder of the 'Everyday Sexism' project, set up for women to record and discuss the sexist attitudes and behaviours they encounter on a daily basis, 'what started as an awareness-raising activity has become a worldwide movement for equality' (Smith, 2015, online). Such hyperbole is misplaced as what we have is a project that conflates the serious with the mundane, the deliberate act with a misunderstanding, and which encourages women to see themselves as victims in need of protection from, somewhat ironically, a state said to be a bastion of male power and privilege. Nevertheless, such 'microaggressions', taken alongside the dangers to our health from the sources cited above, can lead us to believe that the threats to our health, well-being and dignity are ubiquitous, and that a lack of awareness can bring disease and death in its wake. If this is the case then, as one commentator, tongue firmly in cheek, put it 'if there is anything more important than raising awareness, I am not aware of it' (Gutfield, 2011, online).

At face value such campaigns can seem progressive at best, benign at worst. After all, what harm can raising awareness do? However, in reality, there are many problems with today's trend for awareness campaigns that can, irrespective of the wishes of the campaigners, lead them to do more harm than good. One reason for this is that there are just so many of them, each highlighting threats to our health from myriad sources. This drip-drip-drip effect only succeeds in increasing our anxiety as we are encouraged to focus on many things that will not affect us. After all, at the end of the day life may be 100 per cent fatal but we can't die of everything. However, such pernicious effects on people's mental and physical health, resulting, at least in part, from awareness campaigns are merely the personal fallout from what is a more profound political problem.

There are three main aims behind awareness raising-campaigns. First, there is the fundraising aspect to them as they hope to increase charitable donations to their chosen cause. Second, there is an attempt to increase the public's knowledge of the issue in the hope that they will modify their behaviour and in the process reduce the risk of succumbing to ill health (e.g. by reducing alcohol intake, checking for signs of cancer, exercising regularly etc.). Third, there is the positioning of the campaigners themselves whereby it is not just the issue that is advertised but the superior moral status of the campaigner. As Furedi (2013c) puts it:

> The very term 'raising awareness' involves drawing a distinction between those who are enlightened, who are aware of something, and those who are not. It draws attention to the fundamental contrast between those who know and those who are ignorant, between the morally superior and the morally inferior. So someone who allows his children to eat junk food is not only unaware and ignorant; he's also morally questionable.
>
> (Online)

In other words, a clear line is drawn, and constantly highlighted, between the expert knowledge of the 'aware' and the ignorance of the ranks of the 'unaware'. In this respect, far from being political in orientation, the current obsession with raising awareness actually represents the negation of grass roots political action, a retreat from activists engaging with people on the ground, on their own terms, and its replacement with a form of top-down moralising. In addition, when awareness-raising expands from being about empowerment to also being about self, culture and business the cause has to become a brand, but this necessitates being non-threatening by becoming more about product than protest, and in so doing there is a danger that such campaigns become devoid of any 'capacity to articulate or engender any meaningful statement of belief' (Moore, 2010, p. 62).

There has been some debate over the extent to which awareness-raising campaigns can at times seem to be more devoted to fundraising than directly helping the objects of their concern. For example, in relation to 'anti-trafficking' NGOs, Michael Brosowski, of the Blue Dragon Foundation, relates examples of where his organisation has helped individual children in Vietnam and bemoans the lack of direct action from some groups who campaign on the same issue. In response, Tara Dermott, Head of Development at MTV Exit, a 'multimedia initiative to end human trafficking' argues that without groups such as hers raising awareness of the issue little will be done to make the issue a social policy priority. For her, 'it is the role of awareness campaigns to inspire people to care both at a personal level and at the societal level' (Dermott, 2013, online). In other words, it is not a zero-sum game of direct action versus awareness-raising; both can complement each other.

Similar concerns have also been raised in regard to the increasing commercialisation of charitable fundraising, with such concerns acknowledged but seen as a necessary price to pay to increase funds and raise the profile of the campaign. For Dermott, 'campaigns based on in-depth research are able to raise awareness about the issue and provide individuals with direct actions they can take to make a difference' (ibid.). However, the danger is that in order to achieve public recognition campaigns often need to be depoliticised so as to be non-threatening to the status quo.

Wearing awareness

In her illuminating analysis of 'ribbon culture', the growing trend whereby people wear various coloured ribbons (and also wristbands) to show awareness of, or compassion towards, (usually) some social or medical issue, Moore (2010) discusses at length the 'pink ribbon' campaign to promote awareness of breast cancer in women. Often presented as a victory for feminism in that it has brought such an issue into the public and political realm, she notes how its contemporary manifestation actually promotes a very traditional form of femininity:

> After all, the ribbon is a girly pink colour. Less obviously, perhaps, fundraising events tend to involve particularly feminine activities, such as interior design, cake decorating, various types of exercise, and female-only pyjama parties. Breast cancer charities sell bags, lipsticks, chocolates, clothing, earrings, teddy bears, and a whole host of other consumer products meant to appeal specifically to women. In such products, femininity, consumerism, charitable sentiments, and breast cancer awareness coalesce – and it is this strange but powerful alliance that has provided the impetus for the pink ribbon campaign.
>
> (p. 70)

This transformation and presentation of a deadly illness into a schmaltzy form of consumerism and fun socialisation has angered some. However, the growth of such public shows of compassion reveals a more profound crisis of meaning than may be initially apparent. Ribbon culture expresses an existential dilemma for individuals within late modernity who fear both the indistinctness and invisibility inherent within mass consumer culture.

> Spurred on by consumerism, impelled by the discourse of therapeuticism, we are driven to seek out our essential, distinct selves in today's society. However, we are also bound by the underlying knowledge that to find the self we must turn towards others for affirmation.
>
> (Ibid., p. 11)

Due to the fragmentation of the self, its incompleteness due to its inability to achieve 'pure' self-expression, ribbon wearing becomes 'a particularly salient example of how we attempt to traverse the perceived gap between the private, essential self and the social, knowable self' (ibid., p. 11). Ribbon wearing is best conceived as 'a social practice directed towards showing the self to be emotionally expressive and ingenuous' (ibid., p. 6).

The trend to wear your charitable donation on your clothes preceded the symbol of the ribbon or more latterly the various coloured wristbands that we are accustomed to seeing today. For example, Flag Days, when charities give a small flag to wear on a lapel were around at the beginning of the First World War, with the Poppy being launched in the UK by the British Legion in 1921 (although it was initially established in the USA three years earlier). The first ribbon campaign began in the USA when people tied yellow ribbons around trees and wore yellow pins to demonstrate their support for the 52 US embassy workers who had been kidnapped in Iran in December 1979. This symbolic show of support for a cause and a group of people was noticed and developed by some AIDS activists who launched the red aids awareness ribbon at a Broadway show in 1991 with the other high profile use of the ribbon being the aforementioned pink one used by campaign groups to promote awareness of breast cancer (Moore, 2010).

For Moore, the cultural shift from the tying of the ribbon round the old oak tree to the wearing of it on the lapel 'reiterates the movement away from using the ribbon in an act that is ostensibly directed towards recognising, remembering or celebrating a particular loved one, to using the ribbon as an exhibition of the self and the emotions' (ibid., p. 151). Whilst ostensibly about showing awareness she found it unclear what her interviewees' sense of awareness actually consisted of, constituting neither knowledge of the particular cause in question nor entailing any reciprocal relationship with someone who was suffering with the illness or tragedy. Writing 150 years ago, the German sociologist and philosopher Georg Simmel pointed out, in relation to prostitution, that after the physical and monetary transaction has taken place the relationship is quits. Moore (2010) argues that a similar process occurs in the transaction between people and ribbon buying in that it can entail a 'no strings attached' relationship devoid of genuine empathy for others.

The dictionary definition of 'consciousness raising' is 'the attempt to increase people's knowledge of and interest in social and political matters' (Cambridge

Dictionary, online). However, in relation to awareness raising such aspirations are often muted or non-existent. A key difference between the earlier 'consciousness-raising' campaigners and today's awareness-raisers is that whereas those activists who saw themselves as having 'true consciousness' saw their role as spreading the message or, in a process of dialogue and collective action having their own consciousness developed, those who wear ribbons or wristbands are often more interested in showing awareness than spreading it. Moore notes that many wristband and ribbon wearers had little specific knowledge of the charity/illness/issue symbolised by what they were wearing; for some, the choice of which one to wear was made on the basis of which one best matched the clothes they were wearing that day. From a wider sociological perspective, the wearing of a ribbon/wristband was often intended to demonstrate that the wearer was in a state of self-awareness as opposed to being aware of a specific something. In other words, it was an expression of the self, of the wearer's moral status as 'aware', that was being presented for public consumption, a form of 'conspicuous compassion' whereby it is not enough to merely give to charity, you must do so publicly and ostentatiously (West, 2004). Showing awareness becomes an act of self-expression deprived of a political outlook or frame of reference. In this sense it should be no surprise that the focus becomes the survival of the self, not of experiencing life but of surviving it. In this respect, publicly displaying awareness ultimately does not represent the affirmation of life but a desire to avoid death (Moore, 2010).

Such a development is influenced, to a large extent, by the rise of a therapeutic culture whereby showing you care over certain issues has become a dominant social imperative such that a refusal to conform can lead to social condemnation – for example, there was an outcry within certain sections of the media and social commentators when some refused to wear a red poppy on the run up to Remembrance Day. Indeed it is now possible to buy an enamel 'high-fashion' poppy badge; less a reminder of the wartime sacrifice of others than the present day awareness and moral status of the wearer.

Conclusion

The current obsession with 'raising awareness', far from being political in orientation, actually represents the negation of political action and its replacement with a form of top-down moralising within a therapeutic discourse. For some activists, awareness-raising is the contemporary equivalent of the consciousness-raising political action of the 1960s and 1970s. For many on the Left the problem was that the masses, unlike themselves of course, suffered from 'false consciousness', ideology blinding them to the reality of their oppression. Today's campaigners see a lack of awareness as the problem dooming the masses to disease and despair. In each case there is a clear moral line drawn: in the former between those with true and those with false consciousness, in the latter between the aware and the unaware.

Such top-down approaches miss the collective aspect of political consciousness. Yes, people have views that they think are correct and consequently that others with opposing views are wrong, but it is through a process of struggle, argument and reflection that political consciousness is shaped; it is not a unidirectional top-down process from the 'true knowers' to their intellectual and moral inferiors.

There is an idiom popularised by the sociologist Robert Merton called 'the law of unintended consequences'. Whilst unintended consequences can be serendipitous in nature, the phrase is more often used to refer to unforeseen negative outcomes that can result from our actions. The law alerts us to the possibility that, at times, those with the best of intentions are the ones who can do most harm. This is something that many of those behind the ubiquitous 'awareness-raising' campaigns we have today could do with reflecting on.

Presented as progressive in nature, such campaigns usually aim to increase our knowledge of a variety of issues that could cause us harm, in the hope that alongside raising funds for the specific causes we will be better able to confront the problems we face as we go through life. However, far from being progressive or even benign in nature, there are many negative aspects to the current trend of awareness-raising. Far from being benign, the cult of awareness-raising can have a detrimental effect on our health, promote self-expression as opposed to public engagement and is more concerned with the prevention of death than the living of life. In order to combat such a corrosive situation we must, somewhat paradoxically, raise awareness of the dangers of raising awareness. However, this form of awareness-raising will challenge the obsession with the self and promote a climate that can reinvigorate the public and political sphere.

It is not only the above issues that are problematic in relation to awareness-raising campaigns. At a wider social policy level they can lead to a distortion of the true extent of social problems as each campaign group seeks to ensure that their particular cause get as much public and political attention, and money, as possible. In order to do so they frequently publish research that they claim highlights the unacknowledged scale of the problem they are concerned with, although at times the methodological aspect of such 'advocacy research' is far from robust and seems geared to present as skewed a picture as possible. Such a process is highlighted in the next chapter.

6 Advocacy research and social policy

Introduction

Much social policy research today is commissioned, published and publicised by organisations with direct involvement in that particular aspect of policy; for example, the National Society for the Prevention of Cruelty to Children (NSPCC) around children, Age UK around older people, MIND on issues to do with mental health, and so on. Such 'advocacy research', is, in and of itself, not a cause for concern. On the contrary, having a particular interest or passion for an issue can spur people on to highlight social problems and recommend and/or demand interventions in order to alleviate them, often, as we have seen, by 'raising awareness' and empowering the hitherto disempowered. Often, such campaign groups identify gaps in knowledge and commission research that improves our understanding of areas of social concern, which, in turn, can help make people's lives healthier, safer and more rewarding. Even some of advocacy research's most vocal critics (e.g. Gilbert, 1997) acknowledge that it has, at times, helped to raise awareness of hitherto hidden problems and influence social policy in highly progressive ways. An early example of this would be Charles Booth's survey of poverty in London in the 1880s; as such it has a long and often highly noble tradition.

Whilst there is nothing inherently wrong with passionately pursuing an issue that you feel requires attention and rectification, there can be a tendency for passion to override a more sober reading of the acquired data. There is therefore a need 'to be cautious and modest in making empirical claims and passionate and personal in expressing policy views' (Gilbert, 1997, p. 101). For Gilbert, such 'unbiased measurement with committed expression of concern … reflected a standard of advocacy research at its best'. However, he goes on to argue that such a standard has 'steadily eroded since the 1960s' (ibid., p. 103), and that, in many cases, the research carried out by such groups betrays a distinct lack of both caution and modesty.

One reason for this is that in order to get their particular concern up the political agenda, and in the process generate more income, it has been argued that many organisations and campaign groups can inflate the extent of their particular issue of social concern (Gilbert, 1997). For Gilbert, one consequence of this can be that instead of improving knowledge, they can distort our understanding of the real scale of social problems and adversely affect social policy – for example, by public funds and services being allocated disproportionately. The current economic crisis was always likely to exacerbate this situation. As the cuts bite, many groups are struggling to carry on with much reduced budgets, and therefore if they are to survive they need to argue their case as persuasively as possible. In hard times, the harsh reality is that good marketing can make the difference between survival and oblivion for such groups. For example, although the NSPCC's annual report for 2011/2012 shows an income of £135.7 million (90 per cent of which comes from public donations) this represents a reduction of 8.7 per cent on the previous year's income (NSPCC, 2012i). It is not only its public donations that have reduced but those from central and local government also, with the yearly accounts showing that the funding it receives for its 'charitable activities' from government, local authorities and professional groups (for the provision of such things as service level agreements and training) fell from £23.2 million in the period 2009/2010 to £17.1 million in 2010/2011 and to £11.1 million for 2011/2012, representing a 50 per cent reduction in two years (NSPCC, 2011; NSPCC, 2012i).

As such, we have seen many groups staking their claim to be seen as more worthy recipients of government funding or public donations than their counterparts, with one strategy being to publish research which claims to provide compelling evidence as to the scale of the problem they are dealing with, and the effectiveness of their interventions.

In this chapter I wish to detail the way in which this process can occur by a close look at two children's charities, Action for Children and the National Society for the Prevention of Cruelty to Children respectively. This is important as it highlights the unintended consequences that can result from the activities of those who wish to raise awareness with the aim of empowerment.

Moral panics and children

At the time of writing, 2013–2015, the issue of the historical abuse of children is high on the political, media and judicial agenda. Revelations about the sexual abuse of young boys and girls by Jimmy Savile, the late television presenter and disc jockey, prompted a high profile police investigation, Operation Yewtree, into historical cases of sexual abuse that has led to the arrest of several other celebrities who have found themselves accused of sexual assaults against children and young adults that allegedly occurred over the past 40 years.

There is nothing new about societal anxiety being expressed in the form of moral concerns over both the treatment and upbringing of children, often interwoven with concerns over childhood sexuality; Victorian society, for example, frequently experienced such moral panics (Clapton *et al.*, 2013a). However, arguably, since the 1970s such panics and scandals have become a more everpresent feature of British society. These have often involved social workers who have been pilloried for either failing to protect children from serious abuse or murder at the hands of their carers (such as in the case of Baby Peter or Victoria Climbie), or of intervening too readily into the privacy of family life and over-zealously removing children from their parents (such as in Cleveland or Orkney) (Rogowski, 2010). In addition, panics over the predatory paedophile, stranger-danger and familial child abuse have never been too far from the headlines in the past 20–30 years.

In light of this, the current scandal surrounding Jimmy Savile and his activities whilst he worked at the BBC can be seen as merely the latest in a long line of panics over the safety of our children. However, it is the longevity of the panics that for Furedi (2013a) makes the present period different from when Stanley Cohen published his classic book *Folk Devils and Moral Panics* in 1972. Moral panics, as traditionally conceived, were short-lived and tended to evaporate as society worked to restore its moral bearings. However, today, by contrast, there is little moral consensus that contemporary society can cohere around, perhaps with the exception of child abuse, which, in turn, allows child abuse campaigners to carry on their mission convinced in the goodness of their endeavour. In this respect, Furedi (2013a) prefers the term 'moral crusade' to describe the current concern over the safety of children. Furedi's argument is given added weight following the furore that followed the publication of an article in the online magazine *Spiked* that questioned the current fixation with investigating historical allegations of sexual abuse (Hewson, 2013). Following the article's publication, its author, Barbara Hewson, received much media hostility, online abuse and calls for her to be sacked from her job as a barrister. The NSPCC reportedly asked her to revise or retract her article, giving the impression that it is unwilling to have anyone question its version of how society should respond to such issues (Furedi, 2013b). This echoes with Becker's (1963) point about 'moral entrepreneurs' holding on to an absolute ethic that sees the unquestionable truth and goodness in their work. From such a position no dissent can be tolerated.

The NSPCC's advocacy work has been criticised before. In relation to its 'Full Stop' campaign which aimed to stop child abuse, it was accused of making exaggerated claims about the dangers facing children. One Professor of Social Work went so far as to argue that the NSPCC campaign could unwittingly increase the likelihood of children being killed. He stated that,

> While 50 children are murdered each year over 250 are killed in motor accidents. If, as a result of the NSPCC advice, more children ride in cars because their parents won't allow them to walk on the streets then statistically more children will end up being killed in car crashes.
>
> (Pritchard, quoted in Rayner, 1999, online)

Becker (1963) used the term 'moral entrepreneurs' to refer to those who use the media to galvanise public opinion and who have a righteous belief in both their own virtue and of the evil to which their campaign is directed. Cohen (1972) further developed the term in his work on moral panics. A similar term, 'claims makers' (Jenkins, 1992) also refers to individuals and groups who aim to channel public concern around a particular issue, often through a process of 'net-widening' or 'signification spiral' (Cohen, 1972), whereby more and more incidents get viewed as symptomatic of the problem.

Whilst it is legitimate to subject the NSPCC and AFC campaigns to critical scrutiny, it is also important to acknowledge that child maltreatment was an issue in the past and that it remains so today. In this respect children's campaigners do attempt to highlight and alleviate a very real problem. The issue then is not so much as to whether the problem exists but the extent of it and the way it is presented and used. It is in attempting to answer this question that we can begin to discern some problematic tendencies within advocacy research.

How safe are our children?

It is not an easy task to try and quantify the extent of child maltreatment, and the task is exacerbated due to definitions of what constitutes maltreatment varying both culturally and historically. For example, Clapton *et al.* (2013a) cite studies that give rates ranging from 1 per cent to 40 per cent. They also note that such definitional and statistical issues do not prevent writers such as Bolen (2001), from concluding that 'child sexual abuse is of epidemic proportions' (p. 80), although, as I will discuss below, it is more often termed a 'hidden epidemic', the reported rates being often said to be only 'the tip of the iceberg'.

If it is difficult to quantify the dangers posed to our children it follows that it is also difficult to know how safe they are. Nevertheless, that does not preclude the undertaking of research to improve our knowledge as to the true extent of the problem. Indeed, *How Safe Are Our Children?* (Harker *et al.*, 2012) is the title of a research report commissioned and published by the NSPCC. As the title suggests it looks into child safety, but I would suggest that the wording of the title does more than indicate the aim of the report, it also works to call into question the safety of our children. It instils a sense of doubt, a sense of unease, that perhaps, contrary to what we believe, our children are not safe. After all, if they really were safe, why ask the question? However, there is cause for optimism, with the overview to the report stating that,

> In some ways today's children are safer from abuse and neglect than those of previous generations. The child homicide rate is in decline. Fewer children are dying as a result of assault or suicide … and it does appear that the prevalence of child maltreatment is declining in the UK.
>
> (Harker *et al.*, 2012, p. 4)

The report cites official figures that found that child homicides have fallen by 30 per cent, child mortality rates due to assault and undetermined intent have fallen by 63 per cent, and suicides by 16–19-year-olds have reduced by 26 per cent in England and Wales since the early 1980s. This echoes findings from another NSPCC report published a year earlier (Radford *et al.*, 2011), which 'found that the rates of child maltreatment reported by young adults aged 18–24 were lower in 2009 than in 1998' (p. 6). The prevalence of physical violence also reduced significantly between 1998 and 2009 as did 'experience of prolonged verbal aggression at home, school or elsewhere', whilst the figures for 'coercive sexual activity' also indicate a decline (ibid., p. 14).

Such positive developments in children's welfare are welcomed by the NSPCC, but they may, in one respect, cause it a problem. Within social policy there is often fierce competition for limited funds, creating the paradox that 'good news' may not be something that the organisation wishes to significantly publicise. After all, if children really are safer than they've ever been, it could be argued that the NSPCC and similar organisations such as AFC require less government funding and public donations than they currently receive. This is not solely a dilemma for advocacy organisations. As one Director of Social Services said when hearing about encouraging research outcomes, 'I am pleased about the results but don't shout too loud, because if the elected members think we're doing well they will cut the budget' (quoted in Pritchard and Williams, 2010, p. 1715).

However, there are several tactics employed in an attempt to keep the issue of child abuse in the political arena and public consciousness. These include signi-fication spiral and category conflation, hyperbole and the use of metaphor as the findings are offered up for public and media consumption.

Making good news bad: category conflation and signification spiral

As shown above, it is not the case that the NSPCC report fails to acknowledge that rates of child maltreatment have declined. However, whilst such positive developments are welcomed, the discussion does not dwell on them and is quick to move away from the positives to focus on more negative outcomes. The report quickly warns us that there is no room for complacency as the extent of child abuse and neglect remains deeply worrying and 'it is an *outrage* that more than one child a week dies from maltreatment and that one in five children today have experienced serious physical abuse, sexual abuse or severe physical or emotional neglect' (Harker *et al.*, 2013, p. 4, my emphasis). That it is identified as an outrage has the rhetorical effect of foreclosing debate, to criticise would be to defend the outrageous. To prevent us from getting complacent over the threats still faced by our children we are also informed that

> new kinds of threats are emerging, particularly with the increasing amount of time children spend in the digital world. As many as one in four 11 and 12 year olds experience something on a social networking site that bothers them almost every day.
>
> (Ibid.)

In the space of three paragraphs the NSPCC report has gone from admitting that the situation is better than for previous generations, to the claim that 52 children a year die of maltreatment, 20 per cent have experienced maltreatment and that a quarter of 11- and 12-year-olds are 'bothered' by something they see or read online each day. With the more credible hard statistics, such as those showing a decline in child mortality rates, emphasising the positive, the focus moves to more vague and subjective issues to highlight a widespread problem. For example, what does it mean to 'have experienced maltreatment', what does 'bothered by' mean? These are very subjective terms and can conflate the serious with the more mundane aspects of growing up and negotiating a path to adulthood.

The way the term maltreatment is defined is itself indicative of the expansion of the concept of abuse and the conflation of categories. For example, the NSPCC's 2011 report defines maltreatment as

> all forms of physical/and or emotional ill-treatment, sexual abuse, neglect or negligent treatment or other exploitation, resulting in actual or potential harm to the child's health, survival, development or dignity in the context of a relationship of trust or power.
>
> (Radford *et al.*, p. 9)

As Furedi (2013a) notes, such a definition does not differentiate between adult perpetrators of child abuse and the acts of other children. In addition, the definition of emotional abuse is so wide that any parenting strategy of which the NSPCC disapproves can be redefined as a form of maltreatment. From a sociological perspective this can be viewed as an example of signification spiral which leads to the convergence of categories and 'occurs when two or more activities are linked in the process of signification as to implicitly or explicitly draw parallels between them' (Hall *et al.*, 1978, p. 223). The linking of new concerns with pre-existing fears helps to raise the profile of the new campaign. They work alongside the existing narrative of child abuse to gain public and media attention. It is this process that gives vague terms such as 'have experienced maltreatment' and seen or heard something that 'bothers them' their discursive power. In and of themselves they are relatively weak terms, but by being set within a framework of wider notions of child abuse they gain resonance as signifiers of widespread child maltreatment.

A similar process of signification spiral occurs in relation to the way child neglect is defined in the research conducted by Action for Children (AFC). Somewhere between the NSPCC's detailed reports and its media releases (discussed below) there are 'reports' that attempt to summarise research and knowledge in a very accessible way for public consumption, but are often not far short of advertising campaigns on behalf of the respective agencies. Action for Children's February 2010 publication *Neglecting the Issue: Impact, causes and responses to child neglect in the UK* (AFC, 2010a) exemplifies this trend, being another example of advocacy research that is designed more for public and media consumption than to furthering the boundaries of knowledge. It is worth analysing in a little detail.

The report acknowledges that defining child neglect is not an easy thing to do and cites the English government's definition as being:

> The persistent failure to meet a child's basic physical and/or psychological needs, likely to result in the serious impairment of the child's health or development. It may involve a parent or carer failing to provide adequate food, shelter or clothing, failing to protect a child from physical harm or danger, or the failure to ensure access to appropriate medical care or treatment. It may also include neglect of, or unresponsiveness to, a child's basic emotional needs.
>
> (AFC, 2010a, p. 4)

However, in another example of signification spiral AFC argue that child neglect must be viewed in its broadest sense as when a child is not having its needs met in the following aspects of its life: basic daily care (food, clothing, shelter and warmth); safety, health care and stability; emotional warmth; stimulation; guidance and boundaries. On page six, written in red, and placed within a black perimeter with space around it in order for it to stand out, is the following information: 'Studies suggest up to 10 percent of children in the UK experience neglect – that's almost 1.5 million' (ibid., p. 6).

This eye-catching statistic certainly works to draw our attention to the prevalence of child neglect. However, on closer inspection we find that we are not informed what to 'experience neglect' means. No source for the claim is given in the highlighted quote, but in the general text of the report, where the claim is also made, the source is given as coming from the NSPCC's report *Child Abuse and Neglect in the UK Today* (Radford *et al.*, 2011). However, that report asked about lifetime experiences of neglect and also contained a wide array of 'neglectful' situations and/or experiences. For example, following the statement that 'when someone is neglected, it means that the grown-ups in their life didn't take care of them the way they should. They might not get them enough food, take them to the doctor when they are ill, or make sure they have a safe place to stay', it goes on to ask '*At any time* in ([CHILD]'s/your) life, (was [CHILD]/were you) neglected?' or '*At any time* in your life, did (child/you) have to go to school in clothes that were torn, dirty or did not fit because there were no other ones available?' Other signs of neglect given include having a parent who does not help with their child's homework, or who may have left them in the car whilst they popped into a shop (Radford *et al.*, 2011, p. 130, my emphasis).

The headline grabbing figure of 1.5 million children experiencing neglect is not meant to convey to the reader the triviality or infrequency of many aspects of what AFC or the NSPCC classify as neglect, rather the headline grabbing statistic is meant to convey to the reader the gravity of the situation. In addition, no discussion is made of the contested nature of memory. Memory is not replayed like a DVD, it is interpretive, as much influenced by the concerns of the present as the events of the past (Haaken, 2000). Often, it is this complexity of memory, meaning and experience that gets lost when past experiences are uncritically accepted using the frameworks of the present.

Hyperbole and 'startling figures'

The use of hyperbole to gain the reader's attention is a common tactic within advocacy research, given that many such reports also serve as advertisements for the organisations who publish them (Gilbert, 1997). As noted above with the AFC report, the use of eye-catching techniques similar to those employed by advertising agencies is not uncommon. A later AFC report adopts a similar tactic. Written in a larger font than the text on the rest of the page, and in red ink as opposed to the black of the rest of the text, the report informs us that 'Child neglect is the most pervasive form of child abuse in the UK today. It robs children of the childhood they deserve and leaves broken families, dashed aspirations and misery in its wake' (AFC, 2012a, p. 3). This not only serves to situate neglect as a highly prevalent and insidious problem, the consequences are portrayed as severe not only for the children but their wider family. 'Neglect' is given agency, children and their parents reduced to objects, neglect being characterised as a thing that 'robs' children of 'the childhood they deserve'.

It can be difficult not to gain the impression that for many campaigners the extent of the problem is an a priori 'truth' with the research merely serving to confirm their pre-existing beliefs. At times, though, such organisations do admit to being surprised by the results that they find. For example, in February 2010, AFC published a report that aimed to 'raise awareness' of the extent of child neglect in the UK. The report's authors had spoken to a range of people including 'the general public, childcare professionals such as nurses and nursery workers, police, social workers and children themselves' about their knowledge and experiences of child neglect. Analysing the data they state that, '*The results have been startling, even to us.* Child neglect is everywhere' (AFC, 2010a, p. 2, my emphasis). Such rhetoric imbues the report, for example, we are told that we must 'rescue the thousands of children who live with its *devastating effects* every single day' and a response is needed '*urgently*' (AFC, 2010a, p. 2, my emphasis).

According to AFC, the views of children were insufficiently considered in this report and therefore more research was necessary to establish children's views around neglect, something that was addressed by them in a later report published in October 2010. After speaking to over 3,000 8- to 12-year-olds the authors found that, '*The results were startling – even to us.* They suggest that the signs of neglect are rife in classrooms, playgrounds and activity clubs the length and breadth of the country' (AFC, 2010b, p. 2, my emphasis).

Two reports into the same issue published eight months apart both with 'startling results' suggests that maybe the researchers were not as startled as they claim to have been, and that perhaps they would have only been truly startled if their results had found negligible levels of child neglect. However, the same term is favoured due to its rhetorical benefits. Not only are the results startling, but the addition of 'even to us' conveys additional sensationalism to the lay reader. After all, if the results can startle the 'experts' then they should horrify the general public. To not be startled or horrified can be portrayed as an unreasonable and uncaring position.

There is also a tendency to substitute anecdote for rigorous research. For example, AFC's 2012 report titled *Child Neglect in 2011* informs us that 81 per cent of staff within universal services such as primary school teachers, nursery staff and health professionals, 'have come across children that they *suspect* have been neglected' (AFC, 2012a, p. 9). In addition, social workers within the Children and Family Court Advice and Support Service (CAFCASS) are reported as saying that they 'often identify children who are experiencing emotional neglect as a result of parental separation', and that 'staff in youth offending teams in England stated that they can often trace young people's behaviour back to early and current neglect within the home' (p. 10). We are also told that there are high numbers of children experiencing 'borderline neglect' and who therefore fall below the criteria for professional intervention.

However, such figures and claims are as likely to cloud our understanding as they are to enlighten us. For instance, what does 'suspect' mean in this regard, what evidence did they have for this suspicion, and what definition of neglect was being used are obvious questions. It is certainly likely that a parental separation that leads to court proceedings will impact negatively on all involved parties, including the children, but again we are not told how CAFCASS staff defined emotional neglect; did they all use the same definition or did they each work to their own definitional criteria to further compound the subjectivity of assessing neglect? A similar definitional problem arises with the youth offending team's claims, and we are also presented with a very deterministic and simplistic view of childhood. In addition, it could just as easily be said that children considered to be experiencing 'borderline' neglect are children who are not experiencing neglect. This is an issue, for, as one focus group respondent notes, there has been a rise in referrals to the extent that social care agencies can struggle to identify children in the most urgent situations. Encouraging investigations for children not experiencing neglect is unlikely to help such a situation. The manipulation of political and public perception of the scale of a problem runs the risk that we can inadvertently take some things too seriously to the detriment of other more pressing social policy concerns (Cohen, 1972).

Spreading the word: media and metaphor

The ability to generate high media coverage for your particular area of concern is a crucial factor within contemporary political life. If the ability to generate favourable press coverage can make the difference between electoral victory and defeat for political parties (witness the rise of the political party 'spin-doctors'), it can be the difference between survival and oblivion for advocacy groups. Whilst modern communication systems have exacerbated this trend, in and of itself it is not a new development.

For example, Dr Barnado has been accused of doctoring the 'before and after' photographs of the children who came into his shelters in order to maximise publicity and generate public outrage (Clapton *et al.*, 2013a). At this time, the late eighteenth, early nineteenth century, the tactics employed by philanthropists and welfare agencies were designed to shock the public and 'involved lurid descriptions of child imperilment in dens of iniquity and vice, with the sexual element stressed to prick (and pique) the consciences of middle class Britain', and such campaigns did gain much media attention and often influenced policy and statute (ibid., p. 6). For Behlmer, the NSPCC's speciality was 'the orchestration of public concern for the physical well-being of the young' (1982, p. 159).

This acknowledgement of the need to use the media to gain high and favourable press coverage is still evident within today's NSPCC. If the more detailed research provides some sense of balance and perspective with regards to the extent of child maltreatment (methodological issues, signification spiral and category conflation notwithstanding), this is not carried forward into the NSPCC's press releases. For example, a search of the press release page of its website for 2012 found headlines such as:

Nearly a thousand registered child sex abusers reoffended.

(NSPCC, 2012a)

Saville case prompts surge in calls to NSPCC about children suffering sexual abuse right now.

(NSPCC, 2012b)

NSPCC: Babies still at high risk five years after the death of Baby Peter.

(NSPCC, 2012c)

NSPCC warns of child neglect crisis as reports to its helpline double.

(NSPCC, 2012d)

Children who witness family violence more likely to carry a weapon, seriously harm someone or be excluded from school.

(NSPCC, 2012e)

'Sexting' from peers more concerning than 'stranger danger' to young people warns the NSPCC.

(NSPCC, 2012f)

New mums struggling to cope warns NSPCC.

(NSPCC, 2012g)

Such headlines can be interpreted as being intended to give the impression of a significant social problem that requires attention, to inculcate a sense of unease in the general public over the safety of children. They are directed at the public's emotions. It could be argued that such media offerings are of more help to the NSPCC's public profile and income by way of public donations than they are to those concerned with social policy formation regarding children and families or those working on the frontline (such as social workers), or indeed to children themselves. What, for example, do we gain from 'knowing' that 'sexting' is of more concern to young people than stranger danger? The media release is based on a focus group study of only 35 children, but the juxtaposition of both terms not only works to influence public perception towards the view that there is a serious problem with childhood peer to peer text communication. It also uses the public's anxiety over stranger danger, which may equate to 'stranger abduction' in many people's minds, something which is relatively rare and which the vast majority of people will only deal with vicariously via the media, with a more mundane issue, but one which most parents can relate to given the ubiquity of mobile phones and social media. Similarly, the use of the case of Baby Peter in the headline about babies still being at high risk is meant to convey a sense of urgency and imminent tragedy if something is not done.

Also, the figures on re-offending tell us little about recidivism in percentage terms or what the further offences were. Perhaps they were for crimes unrelated to children. We do not know as official figures do not give such detail, and a close reading of the press release finds that it is this that the NSPCC wants to address, calling for a breakdown to be given of the precise crimes committed by registered sex offenders. Nevertheless, the headline gives the impression that a substantial number of children are being put at risk from repeat offenders. Likewise, when the overall picture is one of improvement in childhood deaths, the dramatic headline 'babies still at high risk' drawing on the emotional power of the Baby Peter tragedy is needed to capture the public's attention.

Another common tactic within advocacy research is to inform us that no matter what the research shows, its findings are only 'the tip of the iceberg'. For the NSPCC, the numbers of children identified as being 'groomed' in its report into this area is likely to be 'the tip of the iceberg' (NSPCC, 2012h, p. 3), as are the reported cases of internet and mobile phone abuse, with the hidden part of the iceberg here representing an 'e-safety timebomb' (NSPCC, 2013, online). For AFC the known rates of child neglect are also only 'the tip of the iceberg' (AFC, 2012a, p. 6).

The use of such a metaphor is a powerful rhetorical tool. In essence, 'metaphor is understanding and experiencing one kind of thing in terms of another' (Lakoff and Johnson, 2003, p. 5). As a form of communication, metaphors are intended to create new meaning, to change a person's thinking, to get them to view something in a different way (this is why they are commonly used in counselling and therapy). In addition, metaphorical concepts 'can keep us from focusing on other aspects of the metaphor that are inconsistent' with it (ibid., p. 10). In such a way, 'the tip of the iceberg' metaphor also works to take our attention away from the reductions in child maltreatment and helps to construct a picture of hidden malevolence beneath the more positive messages from the research. In this respect, the 'tip of the iceberg' metaphor not only informs us that most cases of said abuse/neglect are unreported or unknown and therefore need urgent attention, it also implies that beneath the surface appearance of family and community life there is a large hidden sphere within which children are regularly abused.

Conclusion

Contemporary society faces many problems and there is an urgent need to gain accurate information as to the true extent of such problems so that, where necessary, social policy and related provision can be delivered as effectively as possible. Campaigning groups do have an important role to play in highlighting such issues and also in providing services to support people who require emotional or practical assistance. Indeed, a thriving civil society is reliant on people taking an interest in tackling the problems within their communities and wider society.

However, it cannot be denied that many organisations require substantial sums of money and brand profile in order to survive and have some stability; both are prerequisites if they are to help improve knowledge and/or provide practical help to the objects of their concern. As such, attempts to get noticed can lead to problem exaggeration and media manipulation, tactics which may help the organisation survive but can be detrimental to social policy formation as it gets skewed not according to need, but towards those whose benefactors have the best marketing department.

It can also be a way of refusing to make judgements. So, for example, the NSPCC in its broadening out of the definition of child abuse and neglect actually evades responsibility for making specific judgements and decisions and of the accountability that goes with this. If all are potentially abusers and/or abused there is no need to discriminate. This awareness without discrimination has the logical conclusion that we must all be suspect and consequently monitored.

It is clear that advocacy groups do have an impact on social policy but the danger is that the impact can at times be a negative one. For example, in relation to social work Clapton *et al.* (2013b) argue that heightened anxiety over children, as claims makers highlight yet another 'problem' that represents only 'the tip of the iceberg', can lead to social workers being 'unable to discern the difference between genuine and disproportionate concerns' (p. 9). For statutory social workers I do not think this will be a major issue; such workers are all too often left to deal with families suffering the most severe social and emotional problems, and whilst the wilder claims of advocacy groups will certainly do little to alleviate this, they are also unlikely to significantly worsen it.

However, where Clapton *et al.* are correct is in their final conclusion where they warn that 'an ever-expanding list of items on the child protection radar has occluded the growing impoverishment and immiseration of many individuals, families and communities' (Clapton *et al.*, 2013b, p. 9). In this respect, they are also correct to emphasise Cohen's warning that one of the dangers of moral panics is that they can manipulate us 'into taking some things too seriously and other things not seriously enough' (2002, p. xxxv).

The purpose of this chapter's critical analysis of the above documents was to highlight some of the ways in which such reports are constructed and the problems that may accrue from this. As key contemporary examples of publications intended to raise public awareness and influence social policy, such scrutiny is essential if we are to have a more informed debate around social policy and social welfare. Another key area in which the rhetoric of awareness and empowerment, advocacy groups and related research proliferates today is that of public health policy and practice and it is to this that we turn in the next chapter.

7   From public health to personal empowerment

Introduction

Public health has long been a concern of government. In the nineteenth century the influence of the wider environment on the health of the population was highlighted, for example, in the need to improve sewage systems, purify water supplies, improve the quality of housing provision and develop health and safety conditions in the workplace. However, whereas it once was primarily concerned with the control and eradication of communicable diseases it now tends to focus on the prevention of chronic disease and the onset of illness. As a result, the latter decades of the twentieth century and into the new millennium saw greater emphasis on the role of individual lifestyle and behaviour in both the onset and progression of illness and disease, with 'public' health programmes increasingly taking not only a population-based approach but also an individual one. In other words, contemporary health initiatives not only look to make sick people better but to prevent them from falling ill in the first place.

There has been a perceptible shift from social determinants on health to a concern with individual lifestyle, with unhealthy behaviour being the main target of government intervention. This is, in many respects, nothing new; the Labour government's 1976 health White Paper *Prevention and Health: Everybody's business* (DoH, 1976), had a strong emphasis on individual responsibility but this element of health policy has been increasingly emphasised, for example in New Labour's *Saving Lives* (DoH, 1999) and *Choosing Lives* (DoH, 2004). It has been argued that, as these policies have been developed, 'the idea that communities and public/private-sector organizations may also be influential in improving the public health seems to have been abandoned' (King, 2007, p. 96).

This chapter discusses the increasing interest in health promotion in the late twentieth century and into the new millennium. My aim is to highlight the conditions that allowed it to emerge in the form that it did and to discuss some of the consequences of the new public health agenda. As we will see, the above dilemma of social versus individual change and the role of government in negotiating the tension between paternalism and liberalism has been a recurring theme, although as will be shown in this and the following chapter, its articulation has changed significantly over the years.

The rebirth of public health

The period from the 1970s onwards is held by some to have been a key period when there was a revival of interest in public health (e.g. Baggott, 2000; Hunter, 2007). A 1974 report by the then Canadian Health Minister, Marc Lalonde, with its emphasis on the inadequacy of a biomedical model of health care for high-income countries, is often cited as heralding the dawn of a renewed focus on public health (Lalonde, 1974). For Lalonde, there was a need for an upstream policy agenda, one that looked at prevention rather than cure and that acknow-ledged that the greatest benefits in healthcare would come not only from improve-ments in the environment but also by moderating 'risky' lifestyles and behaviours. In the UK there was the *Prevention and Health: Everybody's business* policy document (DHSS, 1976a) alongside the setting of priorities for the health and social services (DHSS, 1976b). At an international level it was the World Health Organisation that took the lead via two specific initiatives, the *Health for All by the Year 2000* and the *Health Promotion Programme* (Parish, 1994).

The changing terrain can be seen in the World Health Organisation's revised definition of health. Whereas the 1948 definition was 'A state of complete phys-ical, mental and social well-being and not merely the absence of disease' (WHO, 1948, online), its 1986 revision now defined health more broadly. It now read:

> To reach a state of complete physical, mental and social well-being, an indi-vidual or group must be able to identify and to realize aspirations, to satisfy needs, and to change or cope with the environment. Health is therefore seen as a resource for everyday life, not the objective of living.
>
> (WHO, 1986, online)

For the WHO, health is therefore a positive concept, one that needs to emphasise social and personal resources as well as physical capacities. Even as the WHO and national governments were formulating their health programmes to acknow-ledge environmental factors on health, there were concerns that health promotion policies, and the professionals charged with implementing them, could be seen as prescribing a particular, 'correct', way to live, and that this could become pre-dominantly individual in focus. This could be seen as endorsing a victim blaming approach as opposed to changing the sociostructural environment as a way to improve the public's health. In this respect, the change of focus away from treat-ment and towards prevention was criticised by some for 'failing to recognise that health is largely created outwith the health care sector' (Parish, 1994, p. 14). In a similar vein it was recognised that the proposals could lead to the individual being predominantly held responsible for her own health and well-being. For example, an early discussion paper explicitly downplayed the socio-economic structural influences on health, stating that:

> many of the current major problems in prevention are related less to man's outside environment than to his own behaviour; what might be termed our

lifestyle. For example, the determination of many to smoke cigarettes in the face of the evidence that it is harmful to health and may well kill them.

(DHSS, 1976a, p. 17)

Nevertheless, whilst the emphasis here is on personal responsibility, elsewhere there is an acknowledgement of a more collective responsibility for health care:

> What is the role of Government in these matters? Is it largely the duty to educate, and to ensure that undue commercial pressures are not placed upon the individual and society? How far is the choice of the individual in these matters a free one and how can the individual be shown clearly the basis for the various options open to him so that he may make his choice with the greatest possible knowledge.

(DHSS, 1976a, p. 17)

For Hunter (2007), whilst this report did not make any specific recommendations it did at least raise the issue of health and a 'prevention is better than cure' approach that paved the way for the first ever health strategy for England, even if it did take a further 16 years for it to come to fruition. Here he is explicitly referring to the 1992 *The Health of the Nation* policy document (DoH, 1992).

Promoting the health of the nation

The Health of the Nation (HOTN) policy was an attempt to have a public discussion about the importance of *health* rather than healthcare. It was implemented by the Conservative government that was in power from 1979 to 1997 and represents something of a paradoxical stance in that this was an administration intent on small government, individual choice and responsibility, and which was not normally seen as espousing the benefits of central planning or the role of the social in health outcomes. The focus of the policy was on five key areas: coronary heart disease and stroke; cancer; mental illness; HIV/AIDS and sexual health; and accidents. The drivers behind the HOTN agenda are complex but one important influence was the World Health Organisation which, in 1984, set out global aspirations for health by the year 2000 and which it revised seven years later (WHO, 1984, 1991).

Whilst generally well received, the HOTN strategy was not without its critics. Most saw the benefits of a health policy that focused on prevention rather than cure, setting out specific targets for cutting mortality rates and reducing risk factors associated with a range of illnesses and diseases. However, the fact that the key responsibility for the delivery of public health initiatives was still located within the NHS was seen as inhibiting the effectiveness of the policy as it would, inevitably, take second place in terms of priority to the care and treatment of those who were currently sick. It was argued that there was a need for a more multisectoral approach to public health to include many of those public agencies who may not see themselves as sitting within the public health sector.

Critics on the political left argued that the strategy failed to pay sufficient attention to the socio-economic determinants of health and thereby side-stepped the need to combat poverty and material inequality. In addition, it was also criticised for still having too strong an emphasis on a disease model of health. Critics on the political right voiced concern over its intrusion into the private sphere of personal and family life and the concomitant moralising tone that was often implied within health promotion discourse. Whilst the critics did have a point about the authoritarian nature of much health promotion polices and practice, on the whole such developments were, if not enthusiastically welcomed, were certainly not rejected by the general public.

The HOTN policy document is seen as a key development in the renewed focus on public health. However, just as we have seen in relation to empowerment, it was the New Labour administration that came to power in 1997 that oversaw an exponential rise in interventions related to improving public health. It appointed Derek Wanless, former chair of the National Westminster Bank, to advise it on future health trends and on the capacity of a publicly funded NHS being able to meet future demand. One key concern he raised was that new health strategies still tended to be focused on acute inpatient care, on treating rather than preventing disease. He advocated greater emphasis on health promotion as a way to reduce demand on the health service (Wanless, 2002), a proposal that the government accepted (Hunter, 2007).

Following the election of a Labour Government in May 1997, the new administration announced that it was to launch a new strategy, *Our Healthier Nation*, that was to be based on a very different philosophy from the previous one, in that 'it would explicitly accept and aim to address the underlying causes of health and disease, and the inequalities in health which result' (Hunter *et al.*, 2000, p. 4). The government had stated its intention to specifically address inequalities in health by improving the health of the poorest sections of society at a faster rate than the wealthier demographic. Assessing the impact of government policy at the time in addressing such structural determinants of health inequalities, Hunter *et al.* (2000) conclude that improvements had been negligible although they did concede that it was early days and therefore it was too soon to judge the results. They agreed with the government that a ten-year period would be necessary before definitive conclusions as to the success or failure of the strategy could be made.

What is most instructive for our purposes is not the details of any specific policy but rather what the debate and associated interventions reveal about wider changes within society. In this regard it is necessary to try to understand the way the Conservative government of 1979–1992, which initially sought to undermine or suppress any suggestion of a link between economic status and differentials in health, gradually came to acknowledge that there was indeed an association. Such political debates and shifts of emphasis over health need to be understood in relation to the wider political climate of the time.

Given its ubiquity today, it is easy to forget that the term 'health promotion' is another recent addition to contemporary discourse, being virtually unheard of until the late 1970s. It would appear that it has had a huge impact on public consciousness. For example, consider the exponential growth of 'health related' commodities. Burrows *et al.* (1994) point out that whereas in the 1960s such items may have included such things as aspirins, TCP, Dettol and plasters, by the 1990s also included were such things as 'food and drink; myriad health promoting pills; private health insurance; membership of sport and health clubs; walking boots; running shoes; cosmetic surgery; shampoo (for "healthy looking hair"); sun oils; psychoanalysis; shell suits; and so on' (p. 2). Their choice to include shell suits is interesting because, whilst originally marketed as sports and exercise apparel, they soon came to be associated with the unhealthy poor via crude comedy caricatures such as Vicky Pollard from the television series *Little Britain*.

According to Tannahill

> health promotion comprises efforts to enhance positive health and prevent ill-health, through the overlapping spheres of health education, prevention, and health promotion. The cardinal principle of health promotion thus defined is *empowerment*. Health education seeks to empower people by providing necessary information and helping people to develop skills.
>
> (Quoted in Seedhouse, 1997, p. 48, my emphasis)

Empowerment is seen by some to be a central component of the philosophy and practice of health promotion. It is said to be, in a similar way to 'health', both a desirable end in itself and also a means to an end; by empowering individuals and communities it will act in an instrumental fashion to facilitate 'healthy' decision-making (Tones, 1997). What is interesting in Tones' account is the way he discusses those to be subject to 'empowerment' as clients who should enter into a contract with the professional as part of the 'behaviour modification' process.

Likewise, Kendall (1998) notes how the discourse of empowerment has pervaded the discourse of health and sees its roots as originating with feminism, the self-help movement and collective consciousness ideologies of the 1970s. However, as it developed the term was also taken up by right-wing conservatism which has facilitated a conceptual shift in the interpretation of empowerment from that of collective to individual responsibility for health and welfare.

Empowerment can also be seen as raising people's awareness in order for them to exercise choice from a more knowledgeable stance. Campaigns to raise expectant or new mothers' awareness of the benefits of breastfeeding could fall into this category, the idea being that with this knowledge the mothers are empowered to make the right choice for them and their babies, and even if the decision is not to breastfeed it is a knowledge-based decision rather than one based on the unquestioning acceptance of social norms.

For Ashton, health promotion contains five principles: it 'actively involves the population in the setting of everyday life rather than focusing on people who are at risk for specific conditions and in contact with medical services'; it 'is directed towards action on the causes of ill-health'; it 'uses many different approaches which combine to improve health, these include education and information, community development and organisation, health advocacy and legislation'; and it 'depends particularly on public participation; health professionals – especially those in Primary Health Care – have an important part to play in nurturing health promotion and enabling it to take place' (quoted in Seedhouse, 1997, p. 38).

Others argue that the distinctive feature of health promotion is the attention it gives to 'the facilitation of healthy lives' by focusing on the social, economic and ecological environment within which they live their lives (Burrows *et al.*, 1994, p. 2). This dual approach of addressing the individual and the structural, although retaining elements of previous health initiatives, is held to represent a new paradigm of health care. From such a perspective, the sociology of health promotion is also a sociology of risk, knowledge, consumption, lifestyle, culture and health.

The moral dimension of health promotion

There are those within health promotion who hold a somewhat fundamentalist view that the ends of improving public health justify the means necessary with which to do so. For them, the idea that individuals have moral autonomy and therefore the right to make their own decisions over how to live their lives, to decide for themselves what is healthy, is barely, if at all, entertained. Often, an apparently objective stance is advocated. For example, in relation to alcohol consumption the evidence base is fairly conclusive that excessive and prolonged alcohol consumption greatly increases the chances of an individual contracting an alcohol-related disease. However, this does not necessarily equate to it being bad for the individual's health. Such a leap depends on an interpretation of health that is not so conducive to the objectivity of medical science. As Seedhouse (1997) points out this involves a judgement on how one thinks life ought to be lived:

> If a person chooses a 'hard living' lifestyle, even if that person becomes diseased as a result, this does not automatically mean that was a bad choice (not if this is the life he genuinely wanted to live). The *causation* of the disease is a matter of evidence or even fact, the *interpretation* of the behaviour that caused the disease depends upon what the interpreter values – that is, it depends on her prejudice.
>
> (p. 79, emphasis in original)

In other words, prejudice cannot be removed from any discussion or policy related to health promotion. It is not possible to promote health or a healthy lifestyle without having a preconceived belief about what constitutes such a lifestyle. Unless you have a belief that one way of living is preferable to another then there is nothing for you to promote. Writing in 1997, Seedhouse noted the growing trend, one that has grown exponentially in the intervening years, from a focus on the prevention of disease to one of 'positive health promotion' or 'well-being'. He perceptively notes that 'once the grounding in disease is lost *all that remains* as health promotion's inspiration are points of view about how people should behave, associate and act towards each other: and this is exactly the stuff of political philosophy' (p. 80, emphasis in original).

The injunction of medical science to show a correlation between certain behaviours and the onset of disease is often a way avoiding moral discussion over what constitutes a good and worthwhile life. Evidence from research may show that abstaining from cigarettes, alcohol and exercise may help prolong your life but it does not provide any evidence that such a lifestyle is the best way for a human being to live their lives (Seedhouse, 1997). So, in essence, when health promoters proclaim against the lifestyles of smokers, drinkers and the unfit they are, in effect, making a moral claim that such lifestyles are wrong. In this respect, health promoters

> would like to think it possible to move from objective knowledge that smoking is bad, for instance, to the objective knowledge that a life of non-smoking – and other moderate behaviours – is objectively good. But the move is really this: the authors believe that a life of moderation is best and have chosen to call this the objective good life – that's all. Unless they had such a firm set of political values in the first place they would be unable to put forward this particular account of health promotion. It is not the objective health concerns which shape their account of the good life, it is their understanding of the good life which shapes what they see as health concerns.
>
> (Ibid., p. 96)

In addition, terms such as 'well-being' and 'good life' in much of the health pro-motion discourse often work as floating signifiers, with little fixed meaning and open to a variety of interpretations depending on the context and the speaker.

Now, there is nothing inherently wrong in holding a view of what constitutes a good and worthwhile life; debates over such permeate moral and political philosophy. The problem here is twofold. One, health promoters often ignore, or fail to see, the moral and political nature of their beliefs and work, and two, when it comes to political strategy, the failure to accord the citizen moral auto-nomy marks a dangerous break with the liberal tradition of the enlightenment and can lead to illiberal and authoritarian consequences.

The decision over what the government targets is also subject to political beliefs, prejudices and no doubt an element of practicality. For example, HOTN prioritised medical issues, in part because they could be more easily measured. However, the focus on other, less individualistic strategies could have been tar-geted instead, for example, improving road safety to reduce deaths through road injuries or the targeting of poor housing and poverty, or other, more social issues that also have a detrimental impact on health and can lead to premature death.

Often top-down health promotion seems to have a patronising view of people who are seen as unthinkingly disregarding their health. However, as some community activists have found out (to the dismay of some of them one assumes) people are, more often than not, well aware of the deleterious impact of things such as poor nutrition, poverty, poor education, unemployment and poverty on their health. What is often forgotten is that such choices are made in the context of the person's life. This was acknowledged by Oakley (1989) in relation to women smoking through pregnancy. It was not that the women were unaware of the health risks but that the decision was taken in the context of the material conditions in which they lived their lives. Similarly, Heath (1995), a GP, was of the opinion that all her patients, whilst fully informed of the dangers of smoking, nevertheless continued to do so 'because they lead lives which are so materially and emotionally constrained that cigarette smoking is one of pitifully few sources of pleasure and relief' (p. 11). Heath argues that rather than an individual victim-blaming approach government measures such as prohibiting the advertising of cigarettes would be more effective in reducing smoking. For her, the 'tidal wave' of health promotion rhetoric, from her position as an inner-city general practitioner, felt more like an elaborate mechanism for victim-blaming. She quotes the poet Shelley who, in 1812, noticed a similar process at work when he wrote 'The rich grind the poor into abjectness, then complain that they are abject' (quoted in Heath, 1995, p. 11). The problem goes deeper than this however. As Wainwright (1996) points out, those who were critical of health promotion strategies such as stress management, counselling for the unemployed and smoking cessation programmes as being a form of victim-blaming are accurate, but they also miss a more fundamental problem in that 'they reinforce his/her low expectations concerning behaviour change' and 'by encouraging the individual to adapt to adverse conditions, to be a "survivor", such initiatives reinforce the belief that any form of social action is unlikely to succeed, that one should simply accept one's alienation' (p. 78).

In the context of people's lives, cigarettes offered relief from stress and gave a form of structure to the day, an 'adult' space where a short break from the children could be taken, all of which gave them some emotional comfort. Davison *et al.* make a similar point:

> The effect of personal behaviour on health is apparently well understood by the vast majority of the population. While this does not necessarily imply that all individuals actually behave in concert with this knowledge, neither does it automatically indicate that repeated applications of the same propaganda would be beneficial.
>
> (1997, p. 30)

A conceptual problem arises when health promoters encounter what has been termed 'outsiders', those who do not subscribe to their way of thinking, people who prioritise the here and now over future health or whose version of what constitutes a good life differs from one devoted to the prevention of disease. At such times it is not uncommon for disdain for the public to manifest or for more coercive measures to be introduced in order to make the 'outsiders' come round to the health promoters' value base. In discussing this dilemma, Seedhouse (1997) points out the contradiction facing health promoters in the case of someone seemingly oblivious to the long-term damage his current lifestyle is doing to his health. The first is to try to improve the individual's health which entails measures to get her to change aspects of her behaviour. The second is to treat the individual as a competent adult, an agent who is aware of the dangers but is willing to run the risk. Interestingly, Seedhouse notes how a simple way out of the dilemma is to ignore the second option, to view the individual as irrational and unaware of her true needs, although he argues that 'it is extremely unlikely that any credible form of health promotion would wish to do this' (p. 111). This may have been the case at the time Seedhouse was writing but, as we shall see in the following chapter, many contemporary health promotion strategies increasingly view the public as incapable of making the 'correct' lifestyle choices.

The acceptance of socio-economic factors on health differentials

We still need to explain the reasons why government policy towards health inequality changed from the 1980s to the 1990s. The Conservative government that was in power from 1979 to 1992 actively sought to suppress or discredit reports that suggested a link between poverty and ill-health such as the *Black Report* (Black, 1980) or Whitehead's (1987) *The Health Divide* that showed that the health of the affluent classes had risen far more than that of the poor in the post-war years. This hostility had changed by the mid-1990s with reports now talking about addressing the issue of variations on health (DoH, 1995).

The highlighting of health differentials based on income and social class inevitably contains within it an implicit critique of the prevailing socio-economic and political establishment. However, such a challenge to government only made sense when there was a political challenge to the current system. The 1970s and 1980s were a period of working class and trade union militancy. Trotsykist organisations such as Militant had an influence, albeit a limited one, within the Labour Party and many local councils (such as the Greater London Council) were under the control of left-wing activists. In such a climate, for the government to concede too much ground over the impact of class differentials on health was not something that could easily be conceded.

However, by the late 1980s and into the 1990s the political climate had changed significantly. Trade union membership and power had waned, perhaps most symbolically with the defeat of the year-long miners' strike of 1984–1985, 'left-wing' local authorities had also had their power curtailed (the Greater London Council was abolished in 1986), the Trotskyist group Militant had been expelled from the Labour Party, and from a wider ideological perspective there had been the collapse of the Soviet Union and concomitant discrediting of radical alternatives to capitalism. The argument made by government that 'There

Is No Alternative' (TINA) to the market economy, often stated but always contested, now seemed to be an uncontested truth. The politics of TINA were transcendent, monetarist polices unopposed.

In this respect the shift in political focus, from one where health inequalities were seen as a political problem for government to one where they could be publicly acknowledged, was influenced, to a significant degree, by the fact that the government was no longer facing any real ideological or organised working-class threat to its political or ideological hegemony. In such conditions it was possible for the government to tone down its opposition to the health inequalities issue and begin to consider appropriating it for its own ends. For Wainwright (1996), these ends were threefold. First, the class struggle in Britain may have been over in political terms, however there remained the problem of governance, of the need for the government to maintain social order. Second, there was the problem of maintaining the conditions necessary for the social reproduction of capital accumulation, which, whilst multi-faceted, necessitated a healthy and compliant workforce. Third, there was a need to reduce the costs of governance and social reproduction, previously addressed by the extension of welfare provision and the powers of the police and legal system, measures now considered unsustainable due to the fiscal crisis. As a result there was a 'need to contain public expenditure and reduce the costs of governance and social reproduction by encouraging the self-regulation and self-surveillance of working-class communities' (Wainwright, 1996, p. 71). It was this, rather than a genuine concern for equity that Wainwright sees as being behind the government's interest in public health. In this respect, the health promotion movement, far from being a social movement was in reality 'a bureaucratic tendency; not a movement against the state, but one within it' (Stevenson and Burke, 1991, p. 282).

Tackling Inequalities in Health: An agenda for action (Benzeval *et al.*, 1995) proposed four levels of policy intervention: 'strengthening individuals'; 'strengthening communities'; 'improving access to essential facilities and services'; and 'encouraging macro economic and cultural change'. Given the evidence base that demonstrated a link between socio-economic issues and variations in health it is interesting, but not surprising, that macro-economic and cultural issues is the last of the four intervention strategies. For Wainwright (1996), the inclusion of the latter comprised little more than 'the articulation of worthy, but rather vague, sentiments', more concerned with political posturing than with any real commitment to redistributive policy initiatives, with reference to macro-economic change merely helping to 'assuage the radical rump of the health inequalities lobby [whilst] the absence of any specific recommendations avoids the possibility of alienating the "realists" in the current administration' (p. 73).

Without more macro solutions the danger was that health education would be reduced to 'blaming the victims' rather than focusing attention on the social and environmental factors which create the unhealthy circumstances in which individual choice is made. In recognition of this, Tones argued for the need for a more radical approach which will seek to bring about social and political change in order to make the healthy choice a more viable option' and in the process hopefully replace the dominant right-wing, individual-focused ideology with a more radical alternative (1997, p. 34). Whilst such a call is admirable, what Tones seems to have missed is that such radical alternatives, lacking any coherent, organised social movement with which to pursue them, were little more than empty rhetoric. Far from being a radical alternative, the dominant politics was that of TINA, there being little sense of any belief in an alternative to free-market capitalism.

The argument that the health promotion agenda was a product of anti-capitalist and environmentalist activists, whilst containing a large element of truth, at least in its earlier manifestations, fails to account for the fact that it was implemented in Britain by a Conservative government. In this respect, Fitzpatrick (2001) notes how the erstwhile radicals of the new public health movement were incorporated into the machinery of the state. Although often criticised by those on the political right as representing a radical and subversive takeover of such institutions, it would be more accurate to see the general result as the abandonment of radical goals and, rather than undermining the system, they unwittingly strengthened it with an infusion of youthful energy. For Fitzpatrick this was exemplified in the way that the Public Health Alliance, a left-wing policy and pressure group, whilst espousing the need for community participation was doing so in a time of decreasing left-wing solidarity. Its 1988 *Charter for Public Health* emphasised things that could not be more different to the individual behaviour change strategies we are familiar with today. It is worth detailing at length its focus on what was needed to provide for the basis of health for all people:

> *Income* which provides the material means to remain healthy; *Homes* that are safe, warm, dry, secure and affordable; *Food* that is safe, nourishing, widely available and affordable; *Transport* that permits accessible, safe travel at reasonable cost and encourages fuel economy and a clean environment; *Work* that is properly rewarded, within or outside of the home, which is worthwhile and free from hazards to health and safety; *Environments* which are protected from dangerous pollution and radiation, and planned to preserve and enhance our quality of life; *Public services* which provide care for those in need, and support for carers; clean, safe water and waste disposal; adequate childcare and recreation facilities; *Education* and information which gave all the necessary information to keep us healthy, and the confidence and resources to tackle the causes of ill health; *Comprehensive health services* properly resourced, free at the point of use and sensitive to our needs; *Equal opportunity* to good health regardless of race, gender, physical ability, age or sexual orientation; *Security* which gives freedom from war, and from the threats of crime and violence; *Social Policy* which recognises the importance of self-fulfilment and supportive social relationships, and promotes these through the provision of domiciliary support and other services.
>
> (Quoted in Secrett and Bullock, 2002, p. 37, emphasis in original)

However, with no grass roots strength, public health professionals were increasingly dependent on the state in order to wield any political, professional or practical influence. In the process, such lofty radical ideals all too soon became subordinated to the pragmatic needs of government health policy. The HOTN strategy then not only revealed the balance of forces determining public health policy but also the limitations of the radical critique:

> The government's interest in the new public health was not in its radical rhetoric, but in the potential of its health promotion policies to provide both a softer image for the Conservative Party and as mechanism for promoting greater individual responsibility for health. Hence it brushed aside calls for redistribution and for action against social causes of ill-health (such as unemployment, poor housing and the tobacco industry) and retained the familiar victim-blaming message of health promotion. Given the wider trends towards greater individuation in society, The Health of the Nation policy was inevitably experienced primarily as a campaign to change individual behaviour.
>
> (Fitzpatrick, 2001, p. 83)

The conception of equality also changed during the 1980s with the demise of the labour movement and working class power. Whereas inequality was traditionally seen as concerned with the distribution of the material resources of society it was gradually transformed into a concern for cultural and psychological equality. This was exemplified by the Commission on Social Justice (CSJ), a Labour affiliated think tank that emphasised the 'equal worth' of all citizens and proclaimed that 'self-respect and equal citizenship demand more than the meeting of basic needs; they demand opportunities and life chances' (CSJ, 1994, p. 18).

Wainwright noted how 'the proposals for intervention at the level of the community and the individual have more to do with the policing (and self-policing) of working-class neighbourhoods and the subordination of critical consciousness, than the pursuit of equity' (1996, p. 81). Although this is predominantly a historical materialist account of the rise of the public health agenda, the relevance of Foucault's concept of governmentality is also clear to see.

Health promotion as governmentality

There are many who use a Foucauldian framework with which to analyse the development of health promotion, in particular in the way it gives rise to an increase in surveillance techniques – for example, in the way parents and children are encouraged to keep diet sheets and those with alcohol problems advised to keep a drinking diary. Whilst these may seem benign, they contribute to the creation of the 'health promoting self' and the monitoring and regulating of the population. We have witnessed a decentring of health whereby health and illness are no longer confined to the clinic, hospital or doctor's surgery but are now dispersed via myriad arenas. In this development health promoters are similar to what Bourdieu (1984) terms 'new cultural intermediaries'.

Drawing on the Foucault inspired work of Rose (1990), in which he analysed the development of the 'psy-complex' and 'technologies of the self', Nettleton and Bunton note that 'health promotion can be seen as one of many forms of contemporary governance which, through the establishment of appropriate social identities forms a crucial dimension of effective social regulation' (1994, p. 53). Of course, it goes further than this in that it is a form of self-regulation as we continually monitor our lifestyles and often discipline our bodies to conform to the prevailing vision of the 'healthy citizen'. This is emphasised by Kelly and Charlton who note the hyper-rationalisation of contemporary health promotion and how it pushes health into the private sphere:

> Whereas once upon a time someone visited a doctor only if they were ill, the health promoter colonises the private world of even the well person, invades their personal life and their sexual, dietary, drinking and tobacco habits, the way they bring up their children, the type of transport they should use to go to work; and provides a rationale for such invasions on the grounds that everything is potentially a health issue! The health promotion philosophy in extremis is much more intrusive in people's lives than ever medicine was. It will even attempt to empower communities when the community had never thought of it themselves.
>
> (1994, p. 88)

In a wide-ranging and perceptive critique of the health promotion agenda and the politicisation of medical interventions Fitzpatrick notes how, contrary to being empowering, the autonomy of the individual is actually compromised as the patient 'has increasingly become the object of medical intervention rather than the subject seeking medical care or treatment' (2001, p. 169). In other words, through the discourse of health promotion governments have been able to regulate not only individual behaviour but also that of whole communities.

This negation of individual subjectivity is also apparent within the debate over whether individual or social forces are the cause of ill health. If some aspects of the medical model of health can be criticised for often individualising social problems, proponents of the social model can be guilty of arguably a more profound problem in that they strip the individual of agency, seeing them as at the mercy of omniscient social forces. As Kelly and Charlton point out, 'the individual is relegated to being nothing more than a system outcome, not a thinking and acting human. The person is the victim of a system' (1994, p. 83). For them, this has the same epistemological standpoint as the medical model it purports to criticise. In the medical model the pathogens of disease are microbes, viruses or cellular malfunction; in the social model they are inadequate housing conditions, poverty, unemployment and powerlessness.

Some radical critics also noted the similarities between the 'healthy cities' projects and the 'community development' programmes developed by the British colonial office in the 1950s to contain potential unrest, and in this respect the healthy cities initiative was a response, at least in part, to the inner-city riots that occurred in the early 1980s in the UK (Peterson and Lupton, 1996).

Of course, governmentality works best when subjects accept the dominant discourse and regulate and discipline themselves. There is no need for overt coercion as discipline is self-imposed. It is when there is a failure to self-regulate in lines with the prevailing health consensus that a more coercive approach by the health promotion industry is unleashed. One of the most striking examples of this is in relation to smoking. Here, not only do we see the imposition of measures to curtail individual choice, we also see some rather disdainful outcomes of such zealotry for those on the receiving end of the good intentions of such paternalists.

Thou shalt not smoke

Interventions by the Conservative government of the 1970s and 1980s to decrease smoking rates within the population tended to focus on educating the public about the health dangers posed by cigarettes (for example, by placing health warnings on cigarette packets) and banning the advertising of tobacco products on television or radio. Little attention was paid to the socio-economic and gender differentials in smoking rates, which showed higher rates amongst women than men, and between social classes (in 2004, 31 per cent of people in manual work smoked compared to 22 per cent in non-manual occupations) (Goddard and Green, 2005).

Smoking was held to be a matter of individual choice, with its attribution to groups mainly used in a pejorative fashion to berate the working class or northerners about their disgusting habits (Carvel, 1987). In this respect the health promotion campaigns achieved success in making a habit that was considered cool and sophisticated in the 1960s into one that now represented social pariah or underclass status. Nevertheless, smoking is a very good example of the way in which, for many campaigners, health promotion can have illiberal and cruel consequences as can be seen with the implementation of the Health Act 2006. On the one hand the goal is to empower us to make the 'correct' choices as exemplified by the title of one government document, *Choosing Health: Making healthy choices easier* (DOH, 2004); the problem is what to do if we fail to make the correct choice, and often the answer is to remove our ability to choose.

The Health Act 2006 banned smoking in 'enclosed public spaces'. The rationale was that smokers can opt to leave the venue and smoke if they wish. They can also smoke at home, just not in certain designated premises. However, for many people, 'home' is also a public space and a workplace and it may also be a place they are not allowed to leave; consider, for example, those individuals confined to psychiatric, residential or nursing care institutions. Many of the patients affected will be detained against their will under the Mental Health Act and therefore may not be allowed to leave the psychiatric unit, let alone the grounds of the hospital. Surveys have found that 70 per cent of psychiatric patients smoke, with around 50 per cent of them heavy smokers, which means that many people deprived of their liberty will also be deprived of a cigarette (Jochelson, 2006).

Working as a mental health social worker from 1995 to 2001, I spent a considerable amount of time on psychiatric wards, and can confirm that the smoking room played a significant role in the 'normal' culture of these environments. Such rooms were frequently smoke-filled, smelly and busy, while the other, cleaner rooms were more or less deserted. Contrary to much lay belief, psychiatric wards are rarely the hub of therapeutic activity or tranquillity. In reality, for those in acute crisis they can be frightening and threatening and, for those more settled, extremely boring places to be. The smoking room is sometimes the only real place where social interaction can occur and where boredom can be alleviated.

Thinking back on that time in practice, I cannot recall any serious discussion with colleagues over the dangers the smoking room posed to the health of either patients or staff. And in my recent or current contact with people involved with mental health user/survivor groups I have had no discussions about the effects of smoking on patient health. Indeed, most psychiatric nursing staff disproved of the ban, with 60 per cent believing that staff should smoke with patients in order to break down barriers and build some therapeutic rapport (a view that was also supported by 78 per cent of patients) (Jochelson, 2006). And as one ex-patient put it, while it is clearly true that smoking is not good for you, giving up may not be a priority when you've just tried to throw yourself under a train or your children have recently been taken into care (Allan, 2007).

One of the most distasteful arguments in favour of banning smoking on psychiatric wards was from those who advocated it on 'anti-discriminatory' grounds. In a reply to the article cited above by the ex-patient protesting about the ban, Louis Appleby, UK national director for mental health, claimed that failure to apply the legislation to psychiatric patients would be to treat them unfairly. Apparently, if 'normal' patients can have a smoke-free environment then 'what message would an exemption for mental health wards send out about the importance of the lives of mental health patients?' (Appleby, 2007, online). Whilst this sounds commendable, Appleby is the 'mental health czar' who supported the introduction of the Mental Health Act 2007, a piece of legislation that introduced community treatment orders for discharged patients and allows for the indefinite hospital detention for some, even if they will gain no medical benefit from it. What message does that give out about the value placed on the lives and rights of mental health patients?

It is also worth remembering that detained patients do not have a discharge date. It is up to psychiatrists, tribunals or the Home Office to decide when they should be let out. Many who live in Britain's Special Hospitals will never be discharged back into the community; others will remain within the confines of the hospital for several years, if not decades. As such, it seems reasonable to allow them to have a smoke; after all, it is hardly going to ruin their lives. Those subject to the mental health system have major parts of their lives controlled by professionals; the introduction of the smoking ban meant they lost control over one more minor aspect of their lives: smoking. Denying psychiatric patients, some of whom will be locked up for years, the small pleasure of having a fag shows how petty and cruel the health promotion crusade can be.

Conclusion

Public health has risen up the political agenda over the past 50 years, from resurgence in the 1970s though to the acceptance of the need to tackle health inequalities during the 1980s and into the 1990s, through to its consolidation as a key aspect of governmental and professional discourse and practice in the new millennium. Nevertheless, how such concerns were articulated developed in interaction with wider social and political developments. In the process the debate over individual autonomy, governmental and professional intervention went from being framed within a context of class and ideological conflict to one that began to take on a more individual and moral tone as wider socio-political issues were seen as beyond radical reform. Change had to be within the politics of TINA.

The politics of health promotion not only gave erstwhile radicals a project with which to follow their political ideals, albeit in a micro fashion, it also allowed the state to connect with the population, something that even health promotion's right-wing critics failed to grasp. As Fitzpatrick noted,

> the key defect of the right-wing critique of health promotion was its failure to grasp the dialectic between the state's resort to health promotion to compensate for its problems of legitimacy and the popular insecurities that had been generated by the social and political trends of the past decade, which found particular expression around issues of health. This interaction, facilitated by compliant doctors and operating through the medium of health promotion, between a state seeking authority and individuals seeking reassurance, provided enormous scope for government intervention in personal life and guaranteed the popularity of such intervention, however inadequate its scientific justification.
>
> (2001, p. 89)

For policymakers and practitioners the challenge was how to turn education into behaviour change. As we will see in the next chapter, behaviour change initiatives have continued to gain momentum. Although frustrated by the refusal of many people to choose a 'healthy lifestyle', there was a subtle shift in policy that endeavoured to use techniques from behavioural economics and psychology to manipulate us into behaving in the 'appropriate way', in what became colloquially known as the politics of nudge.

8 The politics of nudge

Empowerment by subterfuge

Introduction

In 2008, Richard Thaler, Professor of Behavioural Science and Economics, and Cass Sunstein, Professor of Jurisprudence, both at the University of Chicago, USA, published a book called *Nudge: Improving decisions about health, wealth and happiness* (hereafter referred to as *Nudge*). The book has enjoyed tremendous success both in terms of sales and also in the way the ideas within it have met with great interest and approval from politicians in many countries, perhaps most notably in the USA and the UK.

The remarkable success of *Nudge* is surprising in the sense that most academic books are rarely read by many outside the confined sphere of academia, with even fewer generating much public and/or political interest, and *Nudge* is no heavyweight theoretical or intellectual addition to the academic lexicon. It is written in an accessible manner for the non-academic reader, combining insights from behavioural economics and psychology to present a case that favours the development of social and public policies that encourage people to make better life choices. It is an enjoyable and informative read with many examples given of the way in which people often fail to act in ways that would benefit them, and instead exhibit behaviours that will ultimately be detrimental to their welfare. Nevertheless, this alone is insufficient to explain either the book's popularity or its influence on governments and policymakers.

In this chapter I discuss both the theories behind *Nudge* and the way in which they have been taken up by the political classes. As we will see, *Nudge*'s popularity is not due to it offering a new theoretical or political framework with which to understand individual and group behaviour, rather its current popularity reflects a process of the degradation of the radical, emancipatory roots of empowerment. *Nudge* is premised on the assumption of human irrationality and of the need for professional, expert guidance to help the masses negotiate the travails of life. This guidance of human action towards pre-determined governmental goals also entails the danger that public debate over what is the best way for society to develop is bypassed to the detriment of the democratic process. In many respects, *Nudge* represents the contemporary manifestation and articulation of the degradation of the discourse of empowerment.

The politics of nudge

Nudge theory is heavily influenced by academic research from behavioural economics and psychology with the aim being to utilise these theories within social policy and related services. It is based on the recognition that the environment influences people's behaviour and choices, and therefore if the environment is manipulated in certain ways it is possible for policymakers to influence the way people behave and the choices that they make.

There is lots of evidence that such manipulation that aims to influence people's behaviour is very effective, that such 'nudging' – the shaping of environments and desires to cue certain behaviours – does work. Manufacturers spend millions of pounds on advertising, money considered well-spent due to its ability to get us to spend our money on more products than we need and on certain items rather than others. Advertising and the ready availability of consumer products are said to stimulate our automatic, affective system which encourages us to consume more than we need.

The problem for government is that we are often encouraged to behave in ways that are to the detriment of our health and/or welfare – such as smoking cigarettes and drinking alcohol – and whilst we may be all too aware of the long term health risks, our short term behaviour often conflicts with such awareness. The short-term incentives of relaxation and pleasure override the longer-term health implications. Concerned as it is with the deleterious effect of smoking, drinking, overeating and lack of physical exercise on the health of the nation that are attributed to such lifestyle choices, the attraction for government in nudging the population to live healthier lives is obvious.

In a 2010 speech to the Faculty of Public Health, Andrew Lansley, the then Secretary of State for Health, told his audience that

> Behaviour change is the great challenge for health.... The reforms we are bringing will *empower* you – the professionals – to commission services that work – to apply the best technology and the best new insights of social psychology and behavioural economics to achieve real improvements in public health.
>
> (Cabinet Office, 2010, p. 6, my emphasis)

For writers such as Sen (2009) the quest for social justice 'is partly a matter of the gradual formation of behaviour patterns' (p. 68).

The degree to which the scientific effectiveness of such behavioural science techniques has become widely accepted, not only by its adherents within the scientific community but within the wider political and social policy establishment is clear to see. In the USA, the Obama administration appointed Cass Sunstein as the Head of the White House Office of Information and Regulatory Affairs, whilst Richard Thaler was appointed adviser to UK Prime Minister David Cameron's Behavioural Insight Team, more commonly known as the Nudge Unit, which was set up in 2010 following the election of the Conservative/Liberal

Democrat coalition government. The policies promoted by the Behavioural Insight Team are designed to influence our behaviour in such a way that we are more likely to make the 'correct' lifestyle choices, which, in turn, will benefit not only ourselves but wider society in relation to health and lifestyle choices.

According to one government discussion document,

> For policy-makers facing policy challenges such as crime, obesity, or environmental sustainability, behavioural approaches offer a potentially powerful new set of tools. Applying these tools can lead to low cost, low pain ways of 'nudging' citizens – or ourselves – into new ways of acting by going with the grain of how we think and act. This is an important idea at any time, but is especially relevant in a period of fiscal constraint.
>
> (Dolan *et al.*, 2010, p. 7)

This report is titled *Mindspace: Influencing behaviour through public policy*, Mindspace being an acronym for:

> Messenger: we are heavily influenced by who communicates information
> Incentives: our responses to incentives are shaped by predictable mental shortcuts such as strongly avoiding losses
> Norms: we are strongly influenced by what others do
> Defaults: we 'go with the flow' of pre-set options
> Salience: our attention is drawn to what is novel and seems relevant to us
> Priming: our acts are often influenced by sub-conscious cues
> Affect: our emotional associations can powerfully shape our actions
> Commitments: we seek to be consistent with our public promises, and reciprocate acts
> Ego: we act in ways that make us feel better about ourselves
>
> (Ibid., p. 8)

A similar discussion paper, *Applying Behavioural Insight to Health* published by the Cabinet Office (Cabinet Office, 2010) also uses Mindspace to focus on nine areas in which it can be implemented to instigate behaviour change: smoking, organ donation, teenage pregnancy, alcohol, diet and weight, diabetes, food hygiene, physical activity, and social care. The report is heavily influenced by Thaler and Sunstein's *Nudge* to the extent that reading the former often feels like re-reading the latter. According to the report 'most of today's most important policy issues have a strong behavioural component' (p. 4) and urgent action is needed to change our 'National Sickness Service' by preventing, rather than curing, ill-health.

It would, however, be a mistake to view 'nudge politics' as an instigation of the coalition government. All governments, to a greater or lesser extent, take an interest in the behaviour of the population. Indeed, a defining characteristic of power, whether political, cultural or economic, is a concern with shaping and/or manipulating behaviour, and the extent to which this should be allowed has been a central political and philosophical debate for many centuries. However, the rise of the new behaviour change agenda arguably lies with the work of Herbert Simon in the 1940s and 1950s, coming to maturity in the 1970s and 1980s via the work of a new generation of behavioural economists before being picked up and embraced during the 1990s and into the new millennium by the previous Labour administration (Jones *et al.*, 2013). During this period the promotion of behaviour change became an increasingly prominent feature of government policy, in large part influenced by the work of the Labour think tank Demos.

In 1995 Demos published a report, tellingly titled the *Missionary Government Report* (Jupp *et al.*, 1995). As Jones *et al.* point out, this report set in motion two important processes within the early New Labour administration that influenced the rise of the psychological state in the UK:

> (1) it initiated the search for more complex socio-psychological frameworks within which human decision making could be understood;
>
> (2) it suggested that an expanded role for the state could be justified if the more-than-economic drivers of human behaviour could be effectively identified and targeted within public policy design.
>
> (2013, p. 27)

Nine years later, and now forming the government, New Labour's Strategy Report (Halpern *et al.*, 2004), whilst emphasised as a discussion document and not, at that time, government policy, did prove influential, with sections discussing 'theories of behaviour change', 'theory to application' and 'challenges' that could impede their implementation. The 'theory to application' section is interesting in that its focus is on employment, health, crime and anti-social behaviour, schools and education, within 'an over-arching logic' of 'helping people to help themselves'. There is a clear moral message in the report which claims that its approach 'strengthens individual character and moral capacity' by a process of 'tough love' (p. 7). Policies 'must at once *empower* and give choices but at the same time policy should set the default to be in the best interests of individuals and the wider public interest' (p. 60, my emphasis).

The stated need for such techniques is because we do not always act in 'perfectly rational' ways (ibid.). In a similar vein, the Department of Health's Public Health Responsibility Deal unit states that 'Creating the right environment can *empower* and support people to make informed, balanced choices that will help them lead healthier lives' (DoH, no date, online, my emphasis). Such a belief carries with it the assumption that left to their own devices people cannot be trusted; their judgement is impaired, their cognitive system compromised. As a result, we require guidance to be empowered to make better life choices.

Reflexive modernity

It is perhaps no surprise that empowerment began to be seen as a process by which individuals could be 'empowered' to make better choices over the way they lived their lives during the New Labour's period in government from 1997–2008. Tony Blair, the Prime Minister from 1997–2007, was influenced by the theories of the prominent sociologist and political theorist, Anthony Giddens, whose work influenced government thinking and fits neatly with the way empowerment came to be viewed from the mid-1990s onwards. Giddens (1994) notes that for those on the political left the notion of emancipation was a key goal but one that was now joined by life politics and the disputes and struggles that can arise from them. Life politics is about how we should live our lives in a world in which the traditional way of doing things is increasingly contested. It is about identity and choice in a world freed from the old constraints that largely dictated the trajectory of life. Whereas in the past the course of life was largely seen as one directed by fate, today we are said to be free to choose our life path from the myriad available so that the individual has to exercise choice over what they are going to do with their lives.

Developing his concept of reflexive modernity, of the choice-making and reflexive subject, Giddens is keen to point out that such a subject is not primarily focused on the here and now. According to him, 'Where the past has lost its hold, or becomes one "reason" among others for doing what one does, pre-existing habits are only a limited guide to action; while the future, open to numerous "scenarios", becomes of compelling interest' (pp. 92–93). This is similar to Beck's concept of the 'risk society in which 'the not-yet event becomes stimulus for action' (1992, p. 33). For Giddens, we live in a time of 'manufactured uncertainty' whereby the problems we face are largely ones we have created rather than external ones; threats to life such as famine and disease are largely things of the past, in the developed world at least, with the new threats more to do with our lifestyle, in terms of what we eat, smoke, drink, exercise, etc.

This leads Giddens to develop his notion of 'positive welfare'. For him, most welfare systems are designed to cope with problems once they have occurred – for example, the receipt of unemployment benefits in the case of redundancy, medical treatment in the case of ill health. The problem here is that they are focused on external risk and do not attribute any responsibility to those affected. For Giddens, the risks we face are not solely, if at all, caused by external, natural risks but by risks that we can, again solely or in part, prevent from arising in the first place. For example, seeking a cure for cancer is to treat it after it has been contracted. However, if individual lifestyle plays some part in the onset of diseases such as cancer then Giddens approves of 'treatment at source', something that is explicitly embedded in life politics as the 'risky' behaviours are discouraged and the individual encouraged into taking responsibility for her own health.

However, Giddens' approach is not confined to individual lifestyle measures. On the contrary, he also sees the importance of wider political measures – for example, improved car safety and road design and lower speed limits to reduce the rates of death and injury on the roads etc. Nevertheless, for our purposes, it is his focus on the individual choice making reflexive subject that is of particular interest. So, in the example of smoking he sees a role for government in targeting young people to prevent them from taking up the habit – for example, by deglamourizing it, setting up therapeutic groups to encourage smokers to stop, promoting the use of nicotine substitute patches etc. Similar individual behaviour modification techniques could also be used to help reduce the rates of alcohol abuse and heart disease in the population. Echoes of government statements can be heard in his claim that 'social security measures, by and large, do not attribute fault to those who are the recipients of state aid; but by that very token neither do they imply the assumption of responsibilities on the part of those affected' (Giddens, 1994, p. 153).

When Giddens then links the need for reflexive engagement with the potential for empowerment we can see how the term is stripped of any radical notions of personal or collective social transformation and is transformed into one of taking responsibility for individual lifestyle choices by 'not smoking; avoiding undue exposure to the strong sunlight; following certain diets rather than others; avoiding toxic substances at work or in the home; making use of early detection procedures' (ibid., p. 154).

The psychological understanding of, and therapeutic solutions to, problems of welfare are clear to see in Giddens approach. He develops the positive psychology of those such as Seligman (2002) and Csikszentmihalyi (1990), particularly in drawing on the notion of the 'autotelic self'. For Csikszentmihalyi (1997), an autotelic person 'needs few material possessions and little entertainment, comfort, power, or fame because so much of what he or she does is already rewarding' (p. 117). Nurturing this post-material autotelic self is seen by Giddens (1994) as being key to his idea of 'positive welfare' as such a person 'is one with an inner confidence which comes from self-respect, and one where a sense of ontological security, originating in basic trust, allows for the positive appreciation of social difference' (p. 192).

This sees him shift from a focus on material redistribution as the main means of achieving equality to one which emphasises a more internal form of equality by promoting individual happiness and self-esteem, and, as these are things that the affluent would also favour, he sees their promotion as being less divisive than many of the previous approaches that tended to mainly target the poor. The focus is once again on lifestyle change 'on the part of *both* the privileged and the less privileged; and a *wide notion* of welfare, taking the concept away from economic provision for the deprived towards the fostering of the autotelic self' (p. 194, emphasis in original).

At times, Giddens crosses the line between being merely patronising, which is bad enough, to insulting the intelligence of the poor, who are informed that they have more to teach the privileged than vice-versa when it comes to the world of work because 'whatever the hardships they have suffered, [they] have perforce come to have knowledge about a life that doesn't have paid work at its centre or as its main motivating influence' (p. 195). Maybe having paid work more central to their lives is something that the poor would cherish, but in Giddens' post-material vision of positive welfare, how they feel inside gains in importance. The influence on the New Labour government of Giddens' thought is clear to see, the key problem being how to get these reflexive subjects to make the 'correct', state-sanctioned, choices, and this is where nudge comes in and the belief in human rationality goes out.

The cognitively challenged citizen

Nudge is based on the theory that we suffer from cognitive defects, especially when it comes to making decisions. These defects have been classed into four groups: decision-making heuristics and judgement biases; akrasia; endogenous preferences and framing effects; and information problems (Yeung, 2012).

According to the availability heuristic, we tend to assess the likelihood or frequency of risks based on how quickly past instances can be recalled to mind. For example, in the aftermath of a natural disaster, especially if you have experienced it directly, you are more likely to overrate the risk of it happening again; the purchasing of insurance cover following such disasters rises sharply but then declines as memories recede.

The decision-making 'flaw', also known as the 'framing effect', is the one that Thaler and Sunstein rely on the most to state their case. The framing effect describes the way in which how something is presented can influence the choices people make. For example, if asked to choose between medical treatment options in which Option One is presented as having a 70 per cent chance of success, and Option Two which is presented as having a 25 per cent failure rate, many people will opt for Option One, even though Option Two has a higher probability of success (75 per cent compared to the 70 per cent of Option One).

Drawing on research that clearly demonstrates the way in which individuals' preferences are often endogenous in nature, in that they are influenced by the choices of others, *Nudge* proposes that the dissemination of accurate advice can reduce problematic behaviour. For example, by showing how students drink less alcohol than even many students themselves think, publicising such a fact will make students more likely to reduce their own alcohol consumption. Akrasia refers to the state of acting against one's better judgment; I may genuinely wish to eat a healthy meal for lunch, but when I get to the canteen I succumb to temptation and choose the burger and chips rather than the salad.

From such behavioural psychology insights, Thaler and Sunstein (2008) argue that by manipulating the 'choice architecture', by which they mean the environment in which we make choices, it is possible to influence behaviour in ways that are of benefit to people and the economy. In other words, people can be encouraged to make wiser choices than they would otherwise do. Nudge is described as being about 'any aspect of the choice architecture that alters people's behaviour in a predictable way without forbidding any options or significantly changing their economic incentives' (p. 6). For Yeung (2012), the nudges described by Thaler and Sunstein can be roughly classified into three typologies: defaults and actions; physical design; and deliberation tools.

Defaults and actions exploit the tendency for people to make decisions in an unreflective and passive manner, or to 'do nothing'. For example, by having an opt-out clause in relation to enrolment into a company pension scheme as opposed to an opt-out one, it is surmised that more people will contribute to the pension scheme as they will not bother to make the effort to opt-out. Another example, and one that has seen increased discussion in the UK, is in relation to organ donation after our death. Surveys frequently find a far higher percentage of people say they would be willing to donate their organs following their death than actually sign the required donor consent paperwork. In other words, most of us do not take the positive action required to authorise our consent which means that we remain in the negative default position of being non-donors, something that reduces the number of available organs for transplant which can then lead to someone dying due to no organ being available for them. This current situation requires that 'explicit consent' be given to organ donation and has led some to argue that we should move from a policy that requires explicit consent to one where consent is presumed.

Moving the default position from one where we are assumed to be withholding consent unless we opt-in, to one where we are presumed to give consent unless we actively opt-out, would, it is reasonable to assume, increase the pool of available organs for transplant and in the process save many lives. Whilst ostensibly a good idea, such 'presumed' consent may not have been the actual wishes of the person; as in the current situation of opting-in, a substantial number of people would be likely to do nothing irrespective of their true wishes. Because of this, Thaler and Sunstein (2008) prefer what they term 'mandated choice' whereby when applying or renewing something such as a driver's licence you would be required to tick a box stating whether you agree or do not agree to donate your organs after your death. Your application for a driving licence would not be accepted until you had made a choice and your relatives would not have the power to override your decision after your death. Such a policy was implemented by the state of Illinois, USA in 2008 and is the favoured position of the UK Behavioural Insights Team (Cabinet Office, 2010)

Physical design refers to how the manipulation of the environment can improve social behaviour. Thaler and Sunstein (2008) give the example of the men's urinals at Schipol airport in Amsterdam. Concerned with 'spillage' from men urinating, irrespective of written signs asking them to be careful, the urinals had a small fly etched on them. This reduced spillage by 80 per cent as men's aim improved as they used the fly as a target! Deliberation tools can include information campaigns and the introduction of 'cooling off' periods following certain purchases to allow for reflection on the decision, especially if the sale was in part made due to pressure from a persistent salesperson. Road safety can be improved for pedestrians by signs telling them to look left or right at busy junctions. Such interventions are unlikely to be met with objections by anyone but the most hard-line advocate of non-intervention in our right to freely choose.

We can see that many of the interventionist approaches advocated in *Nudge* are more concerned with 'other regarding' decisions aimed at the promotion of collective welfare rather than with improving an individual's 'self-regarding' actions (Yeung, 2012, p. 3). For example, strategies aimed at reducing alcohol consumption may benefit the health of the individual but they also benefit wider society by reducing not only anti-social behaviour but also the burden on health-care services due to alcohol-related illnesses. The fly in the urinals ultimately helps later users who get to use a cleaner, drier, toilet.

Irrespective of whether specific interventions are benign or malign, something that we discuss below, it is important to note that what we are witnessing is the growth of a form of government that increasingly sees its citizens as objects of analysis and manipulation. For Isin (2004), this is a new form of politics that he calls neuropolitics that entails a new form of power – 'neuropower'. He suggests a new concept, 'neuroliberalism' which he describes as a 'rationality of govern-ment that takes as its subject the neurotic citizen – as an object of analysis' (p. 220). If the relationship between the state and the individual is being recast as akin to that between therapist and patient then it should be no surprise to find a paternalistic mode of government develop, something that has attracted much debate.

Libertarian paternalism

Governmental concern with behaviour change is often criticised as state intru-sion into the private realm of personal autonomy. Such a claim is countered by proponents of behaviour change who argue that the government is merely pro-viding triggers and/or support to enable citizens to take greater responsibility for their health and welfare (Dolan *et al.*, 2010). The view of philosophers such as David Hume, who argued that 'all plans of government which suppose great ref-ormation in the manners of mankind are plainly imaginary' is discounted as being sweepingly sceptical and unfounded as, 'there have been many policy suc-cesses in changing behaviour: for example, reducing drink driving, preventing AIDS transmission and increasing seatbelt usage' (ibid., p. 13).

Nevertheless, much criticism of the politics of nudge has focused on its pater-nalistic nature and that it does indeed increase state interference into the lives of citizens. *Nudge*'s supporters do not totally reject the paternalistic accusation but they argue that it is a form of 'soft' or 'libertarian paternalism', in that it does not coerce people into certain behaviours it merely encourages them, often by informing them of the consequences of some choices over others, to choose the most appropriate way of behaving.

Nudge makes two major claims. First, as we have seen, 'that seemingly small features of social situations can have massive effects on people's behaviour; nudges are everywhere, even if we do not see them. Choice architecture, both good and bad, is pervasive and unavoidable, and it greatly affects our decisions', and second, that 'libertarian paternalism is not an oxymoron. Choice architects can preserve freedom of choice while also nudging people in directions that will improve their lives' (Thaler and Sunstein, 2008, p. 253).

In this respect, such initiatives can appeal to both the proponents of govern-ment intervention and those who favour small government. From the perspective of *Nudge*, the state is not telling anyone that they must behave in a certain way (which would draw accusations of authoritarianism), it is merely encouraging them to do so, and individuals still maintain the right to choose or reject such guidance. They may be guided in a certain direction but people can still decide to travel in another direction. In this respect 'to count as a mere nudge, the intervention must be easy and cheap to avoid. Nudges are not mandates. Putting the fruit at eye level counts as a nudge. Banning junk food does not' (Thaler and Sunstein, 2008, p. 6). An example of such thinking permeating government policy can be seen in a Department for Transport Behavioural Insights Toolkit that reiterates Thaler and Sunstein's point by informing us that 'to count as a Nudge, an intervention must be easy, cheap to avoid and should not forbid any choice' (DfT, 2011, p. 29).

Thaler and Sunstein (2008) are at pains to emphasise that they '*are not for bigger government, just for better governance*' (p. 15, emphasis in original). In essence, soft paternalism differentiates between acting voluntarily and knowledgably from acting voluntarily but without full knowledge. The difference between hard and soft libertarianism can be seen by using the philosopher John Stuart Mill's famous example of a man who is about to walk across a damaged bridge:

> If we could not communicate the danger (he speaks only Japanese) a soft paternalist would justify forcibly preventing him from crossing the bridge in order to determine whether he knows about its condition. If he knows, and wants to, say, commit suicide he must be allowed to proceed. A hard paternalist says that, at least sometimes, it may be permissible to prevent him from crossing the bridge even if he knows of its condition. We are entitled to prevent voluntary suicide.
>
> (Stanford Encyclopedia of Philosophy, no date, online)

From Mill's perspective, once the man is made aware of the danger he is free to attempt to cross the bridge. Mill's classical liberal assertion was that the only grounds whereby 'power can be rightfully exercised over any member of a civilized community, against his will, is to prevent harm to others. His own good, either physical or moral, is not a sufficient warrant' (Mill, 2008 [1859], p. 14).

A somewhat similar approach, in relation to long-term health if not imminent suicide, was previously acknowledged within some aspects of government policy. For example, the Department of Health White Paper *Saving Lives: Our Healthier Nation* argues that the role of government is to raise awareness of risk and dangers to health, but 'as long as people are aware of the risk which they are taking, it is their decision whether to put themselves at risk' (DOH, 1999, online).

However, in the intervening years such a principle has come under increasing attack and when such 'expert' sanctioned choice architecture is put in place, those who decide not to follow the favoured path can soon find that the carrot is replaced by the stick. In November 2014, Southampton Hospital announced that the concession for the fast food company Burger King to operate within the hospital would not be renewed. Despite Burger King operating in the foyer of the hospital for the previous twenty years it was now felt by management that its culinary offerings were not conducive to a modern hospital environment (McKeown, 2014). Meanwhile, in December 2014, it was reported that the Clinical Commissioning Group that organises NHS treatment in Devon and Cornwall is considering denying smokers and the morbidly obese routine operations unless they make the appropriate lifestyle changes. Before being considered eligible for non-life-threatening surgery, obese patients will need to lose 5 per cent of their body weight and smokers will need to have abstained for at least eight weeks (Amara, 2014).

Proponents of *Nudge* argue that it is legitimate to attempt to change or steer behaviour in a certain way because, at the end of the day, the individual remains free to continue to reject such influences and continue to smoke, drink and eat unhealthily if they so wish. However, what has also undermined Mills is that we have witnessed the exponential extension of the 'harm principle', both in terms of harm-to-others issues and also harm-to-self issues and also the unification of both aspects of harm. For example, such things as smoking, alcohol consumption and obesity are said not only to harm the individual but also others (e.g. passive smoking, drunken violent behaviour and resultant cost to the economy of treating the health issues said to arise from such behaviours).

In addition, as we live in an increasingly complex world it is argued that people need 'help to manage complexity, to resist temptation, and to avoid being misled by social influences' (Thaler and Sunstein, 2008, p. 259). This quote is in relation to a discussion of the home buying market, and it is certainly the case that the housing and mortgage market can be extremely confusing, so perhaps in such instances some help and advice can be beneficial. Nevertheless, there is also an extremely patronising aspect to the way the need for nudging is presented. As we can see by the other examples cited above, the proponents of *Nudge* not only view us as unable to make informed decisions on our own in relation to major and relatively rare life events such as buying a home, they are of the same opinion of our ability to make the more mundane, everyday life-decisions, such as what to eat, how much to drink, whether to smoke and how much exercise we should take.

In addition, there is often a strong class bias within the behaviour change discourse, with libertarian paternalism presented as a form of 'asymmetric paternalism' by adopting the guiding principle that 'we should design policies that help the least sophisticated people in society while imposing the smallest possible costs on the most sophisticated' and in which 'the costs imposed on the sophisticated are kept close to zero' (Thaler and Sunstein, 2008, p. 249). In a similar vein, lower demographic groups are held to be less cognitively attuned which affects their ability to behave 'appropriately'. For example, in relation to the environment Jones *et al.* (2013) discuss a Sustainable Consumption Roundtable co-ordinated by the Sustainable Development Commission and the National Consumer Council which argued that 'cognitive biases against pro-environmental behaviours may be stronger in low-income families, where short-term concern over household budgets and "making ends meet" makes it more difficult to prompt action on longer-term ecological issues' (p. 140).

The patronising aspects of the behaviour change agenda are often most clearly displayed when it comes to parents, who the 'expert' choice architects clearly believe cannot be left alone to raise their children as they see fit. For example, perturbed by the difficulty of traditional public information campaigns to influence and educate parents of young children, and the low take-up of free parenting classes, a more subtle approach is advocated in an attempt to rectify this, with one recent proposal from the UK Nudge Unit recommending that parenting advice be printed on babies' nappies in order to raise parents' awareness of the benefits for their child's development of verbal interaction. According to David Halpern, Chief Executive Officer of the Nudge Unit, adding a note on the nappy encouraging parents to look up and talk to their baby 'may be just enough to remind parents that every second, a baby's brain develops 700 neural connections and that is a good time to help make those connections stronger' (Hastings, 2014).

As Ellie Lee, Director of the Centre for Parenting Culture, pointed out, the idea that changing a nappy should be reclassified as an educational experience can only serve to guilt trip busy mothers who already have much to deal with (ibid.). She is undoubtedly correct, though from a wider viewpoint it is the disdain with which such policymakers, the choice architects, hold parents that is most odious in such initiatives. The idea that parents do not know to speak to their child unless prompted by a government initiated policy group says more about what the nudgers think of the public than it does about any parent–child relationship.

If some examples of nudge can be said to be helpful, others benign, it is also evident that some are extremely patronising and betray contempt for those subject to them. At heart, we can see a form of elitism within the politics associated with nudge. It is based on the belief that the masses require guidance and censure from their enlightened betters. For example, Thaler and Sunstein's (2008) 'golden rule' involves 'taking steps to help the least sophisticated people while imposing minimal harm on everyone else' (p. 79).

According to Jones *et al.*, whilst 'neoliberalism attempts to subject the state and society to the strictures of economic science, libertarian paternalism embodies a clear desire to psychologise the state and society' (2011, p. 489). They use the term 'neuroliberalism' as a shorthand term to describe the means whereby neoliberal society attempts to sustain itself through neurological means.

> These neurological strategies draw on the collective insights of psychology, behavioural economics, cognitive design and neuroscience in order both to understand the failure of human beings to live up to the rationality assumption, and to correct the behaviour that appears to threaten the future of a market-oriented society.
>
> (p. 50)

Libertarian paternalism is, in part, a response to the failings of neoliberalism and has evolved within a broader climate of psychologisation (McLaughlin, 2012).

For some, it is its location within a psychological state that demarcates libertarian paternalism from neoliberalism.

It is clear that the politics of nudge represents a reframing of the relationship between the citizen and the state. Proponents of *Nudge* view unregulated social influence with disdain, instead relying on an aseptic, bureaucratic view of the universal, of the good, that is arbitrarily drawn up by the state-sponsored architects within the Nudge Unit.

Pushing back against the nudgers

Concerns over the implications of the politics of nudge are often based in moral and philosophical terms. This is not solely over the extent to which nudge policies preserve or undermine individual autonomy and freedom of choice. After all, with the social contract and liberal democracy we already, to a greater or lesser extent depending on our political leanings, accept some form of state coercion in our lives in order for social, political and economic relations to flourish, to stop Hobbes' 'war of all against all'.

Influenced by Isaiah Berlin's differentiation between negative and positive liberty (Berlin, 1969), the debate over nudge often takes the form of an apparent confrontation between two views of liberty, with liberty seen as either intrinsically or instrumentally valuable. From a negative liberty perspective, nudge policies are unethical because they interfere with our right to choose without any external coercion. The government's position is more likely to favour positive liberty, freedom as instrumentally valuable. From this perspective, 'freedom is not valuable for its own sake but only insofar as it is a means of achieving other things we regard as desirable or beneficial' (Zoido-Oses, 2014, online). However, this form of polarisation of the debate between the positive and negative liberty camps tends to miss the real problem with nudge policies which is that 'they pose a threat to the only principle that makes us feel at ease with our acceptance of the state as a coercive power: the right to dissent' (ibid.). This is important when we think that there can be times when how the state views the good life may differ markedly from our own. In addition, having a right to dissent should also allow us to not only

> choose *well* despite the efforts of the state, but also to let the state know of our disagreement. The right to dissent is a safety net for citizens, just as essential for the proper functioning of democratic liberal states as the acceptance of the rule of law is.
>
> (Ibid., emphasis in original)

In this respect the problem with nudge policies is not solely that they are a threat to our autonomy to act badly if we so wish, but more importantly, they are also a threat to our freedom to choose and act well according to our own vision of the good.

For Goodwin (2012), we should reject 'nudge' on three main grounds: first, the concept of liberty on which it rests 'precludes nudge from being empowering in any substantive sense'; second, its paternalistic aspect means that whilst it may not actually constitute a form of coercion, 'nudge seeks to exploit imperfections in human judgement and to this extent it is manipulative'; and third, because 'nudging alone is not an effective strategy for changing behaviour on the kind of scale needed to solve society's major ills' (p. 86).

Goodwin's point about nudge not being particularly empowering is certainly true, but, as we have already explored in detail, contemporary forms of empowerment are also far from being substantive in nature. In fact, I would argue that in many respects the politics of nudge is closely related to contemporary manifestations of empowerment. Also, the contention that nudge does not involve coercion is debateable, especially as it interlinks with other social policies. For example, encouraging people into work has involved getting people to work unpaid with companies for a limited period in the hope that they would then be offered full-time employment. However, it was reported recently that a man who had been made redundant from one firm was then told by the benefits agency to return to work for the same firm on an unpaid basis. When he refused, his benefits were cut (Malik, 2014).

Goodwin's objection is not to the politics of nudge per se but that they are unfair. A more fundamental critique of the libertarian claims of nudge is made by Yeung (2012) who draws on the work of the philosopher Gerard Dworkin. Dworkin suggests that paternalism involves at least three elements: first, it must place some form of restriction on the freedom or autonomy of an agent; second, the restriction must be without the agent's consent; and third, the restriction has the aim of improving, or preventing the decline, of the health or welfare of the agent (Dworkin, 2014, online).

In response to this criticism, Thaler and Sunstein claim that nudge polices are about the promotion of policies that are in accordance with the agent's true self-interest, and also that the nature of the intervention leaves the agent free to reject the choice-architect's preferred outcome. They invoke the philosopher John Rawls' 'publicity principle' (Rawls, 1971) which would prevent governments from adopting policies that it would not be willing to defend publicly.

There are also those who point out that a key problem with *Nudge*'s underlying philosophy is the belief that technocrats and/or scientists understand what people want or desire better than the people themselves. In effect, people are treated not as citizens but as consumers (Farrell and Shalizi, 2011). For Farrell and Shalizi, it is not that advice from experts is problematic per se but that there needs to be more of a dialogue between them and the people, in other words a more democratic process needs to take place. Their argument is informed by the 'diversity trumps ability' theorem, which suggests that 'groups of agents with diverse understandings of the world will solve difficult problems better than narrowly focused groups with higher expertise' (online). They argue that whilst libertarian paternalism is seductive because it appears to offer a way to bypass the messiness of democratic politics, ultimately the latter is better than technocracy at discovering people's real interests and how to advance them. And perhaps more importantly, the more democratic the process, the better the chance of defending such interests in the event of any less than benign bureaucratic machinations. This echoes Arendt's (1970) belief that humans do not only possess the ability to act, but they are able to act in concert. In similar vein, Goodwin (2012) wants to see a more deliberative form of politics emerge. One attempt to introduce such a more deliberative dimension has been to argue that we need to supplant 'nudge' with 'think' or 'steer'.

From 'nudge', to 'think, to 'steer'

In recent years there have been those who have sought to move from 'nudge' to 'think', mainly in an effort to overcome the weakness of the former in its bypassing of deliberative democracy. 'Think' shares with 'nudge' the view that people are rational but that this is a 'bounded rationality' due to cognitive limitations and the tendency to make some decisions based on rules of thumb, habits and emotions.

Nudge, as discussed above, at its most basic is about giving people information and social cues by arranging the environment in certain ways. In short, it downplays human reasoning and discourages thinking. In response to this, John *et al.* (2013) argue that 'it is possible to get citizens to *think* through challenging issues in innovative ways that allow for evidence, and the opinions of all, to count' (p. 10, my emphasis). 'Think' as an alternative means of transforming civic behaviour is influenced by Habermas' (1984) work on communicative action, being primarily concerned with reinvigorating deliberative democracy and its overriding principle that 'the legitimacy of politics rests on public deliberation between free and equal citizens' (John *et al.*, 2013, p. 11). For John *et al.* 'Deliberative democrats provide a clear account of civic behaviour: under deliberative conditions citizens' behaviour is shaped in a more civic orientation as they consider the views and perspectives of others' (p. 10).

John *et al.* see such a process of civic engagement as being reliant on institutional measures that create safe spaces in which citizens can deliberate, and also that the participants have to have a belief that their views and opinions will have a meaningful influence on political decision-making. The lack of citizen engagement in the political process today is held to be, at least in part, due to current governmental institutions failing on this latter point.

'Think' also differs from 'nudge' in that the latter sees the state 'as educator and the role of the policy-maker as paternalistic expert, steering citizens down paths that are more beneficial to them and society at large' (ibid., p. 18). Citizens are seen as being who or what they are, with the nudger guiding their unconscious towards making better decisions. In contrast to this, 'think' is said to have a more optimistic belief in human decision-making, the individual being viewed as able to step out of her day-to-day experience, consider other perspectives, and, via discussion and debate, reach better decisions.

'Think' is therefore said to offer transparency as opposed to the behind closed doors machinations of nudge politics. John *et al.* make the same point as Thaler and Sunstein regarding there being no neutral position, either in a natural or moral sense. Individual decision-making is already influenced by such things as commercial advertising, peer pressure, social values and cultural norms. There is no neutral position; non-intervention is said to merely endorse the current situation. For example, in relation to the location of high street betting shops it is clear that there is a spatial targeting by the gambling industry of certain communities (e.g. areas with high unemployment, mental health problems etc. whose inhabitants are said to be more prone to use betting shops). In other words, the gambling industry is creating a choice architecture that encourages (nudges) people to gamble. Policy-makers, therefore, are said to be merely additional choice architects amongst many pre-existing others. Such is the power being given to such policy executives and 'choice architects' via the discourse of psychology and neurology that they have been dubbed 'psychocrats' (Jones *et al.*, 2013, p. 51).

In addition, the politicians have a crucial advantage in terms of moral authority in that they can be said to have a mandate from the electorate. So, by inviting citizens into more civic and democratic deliberation forums 'think' can be seen as an improvement on nudge. However, the claims and involvement of the public in debate and decision-making for 'think' as advocated by John *et al.* are overstated and, in many respects, suffer from similar problems as the strategies of empowerment that we discussed earlier.

A key criticism of *Nudge* is the way in which it can bypass public discussion. It favours a form of public engagement that 'tends only to occur once the policy initiative has been developed, and tends to close off the possibility for effective deliberation on the ethics and efficacy of the policy' (Jones *et al.*, 2013, p. 47). Whilst 'think' purports to overcome this problem of democratic accountability, the format it proposes is itself very limited. The issues and options up for discussion are mostly pre-set prior to any public discussion. In other words the parameters of the discussion, the list of policy options to choose from are likely to have already been decided behind closed doors away from public scrutiny. The choices we have are therefore akin to a pre-selected menu, often made up of items that favour behaviours most beneficial to a capitalist market economy. In addition, we are in effect talking about focus groups in relation to policy discussions, a self-selected group who have not been mandated by the wider public and who will be unlikely to represent the interests of the wider community.

In terms of pre-set policies taken as an a priori good, John *et al.* (2013) have a chapter looking at the most effective ways to get people to recycle. Here, recycling is seen as an unquestioned good in its own right. However, it can be argued that such an individual response to household waste is ineffective and insignificant compared to more industrial pollutants. Strategies to increase the number of people voting in elections are discussed in another chapter. Again, it is possible to argue that the decrease in voter turnout at election times has more to do with the lack of alternative policies by the mainstream parties, and a significant proportion of the electorate feeling a sense of estrangement from both the political establishment and the democratic process, than it has with public apathy. In this instance it could be argued that it is the political parties that need to change their behaviour rather than the non-voting citizens.

In addition to 'nudge' and 'think', a further initiative, 'steer', has been proposed by the Royal Society for the Encouragement of Arts, Manufactures and Commerce (RSA) which is influenced by developments in neuroscience and the social nature of the brain. In similar vein to 'think' it favours deliberation using the principles of behavioural psychology and neuroscience but believes that subjects require to be steered into more socially responsible ways.

The RSA's director is Mathew Taylor, former chief policy advisor to Tony Blair when he was the UK Prime Minister. Taylor published an article in *Prospect* magazine, a relatively influential journal within UK social policy circles, in which he claimed that insights from behavioural neuroscience could help explain why conservatives and social democrats apparently draw on different aspects of human incentives (Taylor, 2009).

With such a background it is no surprise to find that 'steer' is influenced by Giddens' concept of reflexive modernity, which sought to understand the human condition in a globalised world shorn of tradition and beset with myriad risks. It is hoped that Steer can help traverse the traditional left/right political dichotomy towards something similar to Giddens' 'third way' of political theory that attempted to get beyond the old left/right political ideological divide (Giddens, 2000).

According to Steer, 'it is neurologically reflexive citizens, not choice architects or policy evaluators, who are the experts of their own brains and behaviour – although this expertise is mediated by workshop facilitators' (Jones *et al.*, 2013, p. 180), although I would replace the word 'mediated' for 'directed' as the agenda is set to follow a pre-determined policy or behavioural goal.

The weakness of neuroscientific explanations for human behaviour has been highlighted by Ray Tallis who argues that they forget that our consciousness is *not* located *in* the brain. On the contrary our sense of the world is made via 'a network of significances upheld by the *community of minds* of which we individually are only a part' (Tallis, 2011, p. 93, my emphasis). In other words, our consciousness is a collective endeavour and not obtained at the level of individual neurology. For Tallis, the claims made on behalf of neuroscience by its proponents are often exaggerated and/or offered up to the public via the media in such a way that instead of neuroscience we get a form of what he calls 'neuromania'. Such concerns highlight the need for caution in approaching the intersection of neuroscience and public policy.

Conclusion

In Chapter 2 we considered Foucault's influential work on governmentality and psychological power. His insights have been utilised in analyses of the behaviour change agenda (e.g. Jones *et al.*, 2011 and others).

In their detailed critique of the behaviour change agenda, Jones *et al.* (2013) argue that what unites 'nudge', 'think' and 'steer' is that they all start 'with a universal theory of the human subject'; in the case of 'steer' 'the neurologically reflexive, transformative person' on which 'the schema for behaviour change is based'. As such, neither can 'help us to understand the power relations which must necessarily underpin the formation of this subject, nor provide us with the conceptual apparatus needed to be critically reflexive towards the way we come to see ourselves as we do' (pp. 181–182). To do so, for them, necessitates a return to Foucault and his distinctive approach to power. For Jones *et al.* (2011), analysing the rise of libertarian paternalism via a Foucauldian framework of governmentality offers three critical insights: first, it stresses the necessity to critically investigate 'the rationalities that are used to justify particular forms and styles of government' (p. 490); second, an analysis of the connection between knowledge and power; and third, critical attention to the 'epistemological violence that is carried out when government is conducted at aggregate scales' so that strategies to govern the collective psyche are established but at such a distance that little consideration is given to how they may impact on different psychological subjects (p. 491).

Jones *et al.* correctly note that in many ways Foucault's work, whilst seemingly mainly concerned with the workings of power, was primarily about the formation of the subject. In relation to the way the behaviour change agenda is discussed via 'nudge', 'think' and 'steer' they also correctly note that sociological, cultural and political analyses are marginalised. However, whilst they make a much needed contribution to the debate they themselves fail to detail some important wider social and political developments that have impacted on the behaviour change agenda and on the degraded view of the subject today. Likewise, they perceptively note that within the philosophy of 'steer' 'empowerment is to be achieved not by changing the world, but by changing the self' (p. 181), with self-knowledge being prioritised over knowledge of the external world.[1] Nevertheless, this is to forget that the focus on the self has been the trajectory of empowerment long before 'steer' came along.

To understand the behaviour change agenda and the workings of power certainly requires an engagement with the work of Foucault, but it also necessitates an understanding of the way in which his work was picked up by many political activists and how their focus on micropower and interpersonal relations helped lay the ground for the behaviour change agenda currently in vogue. So whilst it is correct to identify the crisis of neoliberalism as being a key factor in the rise of behaviour change initiatives, the drivers are far wider than many acknowledge. The collapse of alternatives to capitalism saw many former radicals eschew wider political change in favour of more micro approaches, and if 'the personal is political', as many feminists proclaimed, then the site for political action can become focused on the self. The rise of diversity awareness training, codes of conduct and the policing of language, many of which were demanded by self-proclaimed progressives, are but the other side of the neoliberal behaviour change agenda.

The behaviour change agenda, in whatever guise, ultimately rests on the belief by its proponents that the public cannot discuss, debate and deliberate in order to achieve a conception of the good life and that general interests cannot arise organically from civil society, and so, whether by 'nudge', 'think' or 'steer' it is the state that is to decide, in a somewhat arbitrary and bureaucratic manner, the way in which we should live our lives.

Note

1 The influence of Martin Seligman's 'positive psychology' is apparent in much of this debate (see Seligman and Csikszentmihalyi (2000) for a brief introduction to the topic).

Conclusion

The subject of empowerment

The goal of empowerment is often seen as one that expresses a positive vision of the human subject, a process that can help unlock the human potential and thereby enable people to take more control over their lives. Empowering others is therefore presented as a way of allowing people to overcome barriers to their development and become more able to achieve their ambitions. In this respect it could be seen as extending the liberal project of modernity in that it is concerned with increasing the realm of human freedom. From the perspective of the 'empowerers', those who seek to use their skills to help others develop theirs, by giving people, or helping them develop, such things as skills, advice and information they empower them to make better, more informed decisions. The subjects of empowerment strategies may still make an unwise choice but at least they do so from a position of knowledge rather than one of ignorance about the issues involved.

However, this tendency to place the human subject or agent at the centre of intervention, whilst often portrayed as being human-centred and empowering, misses the point that

> focusing on the inculcation of individual and community agency, ethical reflexivity or resilience, as a way of addressing problems of insecurity, conflict or development, tends to see the human subject as the problem, rather than the material social and economic relations within which it is embedded.
>
> (Chandler, 2013, p. 1)

In other words, the focus on individual agency tends to see the solution to such problems as resolvable via the behaviour modification of those subject to intervention; the paradox is that whilst human agency is seen as the solution, the human subject is presented as the problem, as that which requires modification. Whilst Chandler's analysis is concerned with the sphere of international relations, his main thesis is pertinent to the whole debate around empowerment. Concerned with increasing human freedom and autonomy, those who seek to empower others conceptualise human freedom at the level of individual behaviour. In this respect, such approaches actually limit the scope for social transformation because the problems are located in the behaviour and decisions of those individuals held to require empowering. The focus tends to be an internal one that prioritises the inner-world of the subject or narrowly circumscribed community rather than the wider external world of political, economic or structural change.

In the framework of empowerment the freedom of the subject is recast in a negative light, as something that requires to be 'empowered', 'made aware' or 'educated' in order that the subject can exercise his or her freedom in the correct manner. Today, as we have seen, many policymakers, campaign groups and activists are concerned that the subject will choose the wrong course of action whether this is in relation to the environment, personal health, choice of elected representatives or child-rearing practices.

The contemporary subject is seen as irrational and not to be trusted to make decisions on its own. In this sense the freedom said to be achieved through the strategy of empowerment, with its focus on inculcating the correct choice-making behaviour by emphasising the adverse repercussions of making the wrong choices, is not real freedom at all. The agent-centred approach advocated by government is no longer about being responsible for the material provision of life's necessities but about enabling the development of the populace's reasoning capacity. In other words, the focus is on changing the internal cognitive processes of individuals in order that they will make the 'correct' choices in their everyday life.

Individual choice-making also carries grave consequences if the wrong choice is made. For example, parental choice is accorded great significance with regard to children; breast-feeding, reading, 'quality' time, lack of affection in the early years, parental smoking etc. are all said to impact negatively on children's emotional and intellectual development. How you parent then is not a matter of free parental choice, of following your instinct, it is transformed into one of necessity due to the potential repercussions of making the 'wrong' choice.

My main contention has been that the current articulation of power and empowerment is historically specific and has been influenced by many developments; hence my emphasis has been on the interaction between social theory, social policy and political change. As we have seen, in its earlier manifestations the goal of empowerment was connected to the struggle for equality by oppressed groups and contained within it an explicit critique of prevailing social conditions and relations of power. For the more radical elements of these movements, empowerment was more about seizing power than getting it via the benevolence of government, social worker or health professional. With the demise of the movements from which the radical roots of empowerment emerged, the term itself began to change. As we saw in Chapter 4, as the term began to permeate social work discourse it played a role in ostensibly creating a more equal relationship between professional and client whilst simultaneously drawing the client into processes of governance over which, in reality, her control was severely limited. A similar process was also apparent in the changing focus within health promotion, where the initial reluctance by government to acknowledge a link between poverty and ill health was, at least in part, due to such a link containing an implicit critique of capitalist social relations. At a time of widespread class conflict and ideological challenge, to acknowledge such health differentials was considered too risky a strategy. Once such a threat had receded it became possible for government to concede the argument, and, with the help of many erstwhile radicals, implement policies and interventions with the goal of tackling health inequalities and improving the health of the nation. However, such policies adopted a more individual focus and contained a moral-istic element to them that was markedly different to the earlier radical demands for measures to combat health inequality which highlighted more macro struc-tural issues that adversely affected the health of the poor. The reluctance to acknowledge the impact of poverty on ill-health was, at least in part, due to a fear of the masses, of an organised working class with an ideological cause to sustain it, challenging the prevailing social system. Now that this threat has lost its potency, the fear is no longer there but it has been replaced by a disdain for the masses.

The vacuum left by the demise of the larger social movements based on such issues as class, gender and race has also allowed the public and political sphere to be increasingly dominated by smaller campaigning organisations that, whilst claiming to work on behalf of some group or another, lack any social base within the group they claim to represent. In seeking to empower their group of choice, such organisations often make a valuable contribution to society by increasing our knowledge of hitherto unknown or under-acknowledged social problems. Nevertheless, as we saw in Chapter 6, this is not always the case and often such advocacy groups can distort social policy as they use questionable tactics in order to ensure their particular concern rises within public and political dis-course. The aim is awareness-raising, a goal that is markedly different from the previous endeavours of political activists who sought to engage in struggle, con-front social and political problems and develop a more radical, political consciousness.

A common criticism of contemporary political ideology is that it is too indi-vidualistic in nature, with little social analysis of the cause of personal and social problems. Whilst there is certainly some truth in this, it is not the case that gov-ernmental rhetoric or practice places the individual subject centre-stage, respons-ible for forging her way in the world. On the contrary, as we have seen, the individual is seen as cognitively challenged, in need of nudging or steering in the 'correct' direction. As strange and counter-intuitive as it may seem, if we wish to create a *society* we must first uphold the principle of individual autonomy. In so doing we can challenge the view of us as being 'cognitively-impaired' and in need of behaviour change techniques implemented by our 'betters'.

Empowerment as a term is so ingrained within policy and public discourse today and used in such diverse ways that it can at times seem that it can mean whatever its proponents wish it to be. However, such ubiquity of meaning renders the term meaningless as a signifier; if it can mean anything then it means nothing. In this respect, whilst I have subjected the term to critical analysis throughout the book, there is nothing to be gained by automatically rejecting or embracing the term whenever one comes across it. From its radical roots through to its more micro manifestations within social work and social care, much good work has been done in its name, whether that has been in raising the political consciousness of the oppressed in the struggle for social change or in developing the strengths, social support and necessary resources to allow vulnerable individuals to gain a greater degree of control over their lives.

Many people require help from health or social care agencies at various points in their lives, some require professional input throughout their lives in order to allow them to function in as best a way as possible. In acknowledging this, it is the actions and outcomes that need to be evaluated: who is being empowered and why. Increasingly it is the whole populace that is seen as in need of professional help, subject to behaviour change techniques as we are nudged into adopting the requisite standard of behaviour. The individual focus of such interventions is held by many to be the key problem with them in that they downplay or ignore wider socio-economic influences on the health and well-being of individuals.

However, in attacking individualism such critics share much in common with those whom they purport to disagree with. Those behind the behaviour change agenda, whether in government, health or social policy circles, despite the rhetoric of individual choice and responsibility, harbour a distrust of the actual individual's ability to make an appropriate choice. Nudge, steer, awareness-raising, and health promotion all take as their starting point the need to improve the decision-making powers of the cognitively impaired citizen. This differs from the use of empowerment as a vehicle to improve the lives of those who, for a variety of reasons, do require professional support. The current emphasis views us all through the prism of cognitive impairment.

We discussed the ordeals of the subject in Chapter 2, specifically focusing on the decentring of the subject within much postmodern thought. Presented as a radical decentring, it called into question the liberal concept of the autonomous subject in order to understand the processes and social influences on subject formation. However, in highlighting that subject formation does not occur in a vacuum, it is easy to forget that neither did such theoretical developments take place outside society. What has been termed the 'death of the subject' was the result of historical, material and theoretical interaction. The evolution of social policy and concerns over individual behaviour likewise cannot be isolated from such a process of change. Indeed, as we saw in Chapter 7, former radicals, influenced by postmodern critiques of the subject, played a key part in the implementation of the behaviour change agenda. Initially seen as a way of pursuing political goals in a period of declining class consciousness, such initiatives soon lost any radical kernel and became institutionalised within government circles as a moral imperative with which to berate the masses.

In this respect, the change from consciousness-raising to awareness-raising is more than one of semantic detail. Whereas the latter contained a belief in the ability of grassroots solidarity and struggle as a vehicle for the development of the subject (the notion of false-consciousness notwithstanding), the latter involves a top-down approach whereby the enlightened inform the rest of us how best to live our lives.

The permeation of empowerment into social and political discourse is something that took me by surprise as I began researching for this book. I was acutely aware of its ubiquity within social work circles, indeed charting such a development was a key aim of mine. What took me by surprise was the myriad fields within which empowerment was utilised as a form of social policy intervention. It transpired that social work, arguably a profession in which empowerment has something of a role, albeit one not without contradictions, is but one aspect of the empowerment agenda.

Many have, rightly in my opinion, criticised Foucault for decentring the subject to such an extent that he has, however inadvertently, helped influence a situation in which the individual is seen as suspect, and that in focusing too much on the micro workings of power he downplays the power of the state in contemporary society, although more often than not it is those influenced by him who look to the state to manage the micro-sphere of human interaction. However, his notion of governmentality is worthy of more attention than it often gets. We can utilise his micro analysis of the workings of power to highlight the way in which macro institutions such as the state and its proxies attempt to both police and change our behaviour. The radical roots of empowerment are long gone, its descendants a compilation of members of government, health and social care professionals, advocacy groups and awareness-raisers. To reclaim real power and control over our lives we need to critically scrutinise both the concept and practice of empowerment.

References

Adams, R. (1990) *Self-Help, Social Work and Empowerment*, London: Macmillan.

Adams, R. (2008) *Empowerment, Participation and Social Work*, 4th edition, Hampshire: Palgrave.

Adewunmi, B. (2014) 'Kimberlé Crenshaw on Intersectionality: "I wanted to come up with an everyday metaphor that anyone could use"', *The New Statesman*, 2 April 2014. Available online at www.newstatesman.com/lifestyle/2014/04/kimberl-crenshaw-intersectionality-i-wanted-come-everyday-metaphor-anyone-could (accessed on 7 February 2015).

AFC (2010a) (Action for Children) 'Neglecting the Issue: Impact, causes and responses to child neglect in the UK', Action for Children. Available online at www.actionforchildren.org.uk/media/926937/neglecting_the_issue.pdf (accessed on 12 July 2012).

AFC (2010b) (Action for Children) 'Seen and Now Heard: Taking action on child neglect', Action for Children. Available online at www.actionforchildren.org.uk/media/52188/seen_and_now_heard_-_child_neglect_report.pdf (accessed on 12 July 2012).

AFC (2012a) (Action for Children) 'Child Neglect in 2011: An annual review by Action for Children in partnership with the University of Stirling', Action for Children. Available online at www.actionforchildren.org.uk/media/2760817/childneglectin2011.pdf (accessed on 12 July 2012).

AFC (2012b) 'Payday Lenders Targeting Vulnerable Families this Christmas'. Available online at www.actionforchildren.org.uk/news/archive/2012/november/payday-lenders-targetting-vulnerable-families-this-christmas (accessed on 15 May 2013).

AHRC (2001) (Australian Human Rights Commission) 'Gender and Race Intersectionality'. Available online at www.humanrights.gov.au/hreoc-website-racial-discrimination-national-consultations-racism-and-civil-society-0 (accessed on 21 January 2015).

Aitkenhead, D. (2012) 'Stella Creasy: "You can see a perfect storm coming"', *Guardian*. Available online at www.theguardian.com/politics/2012/apr/08/stella-creasy-perfect-storm-coming (accessed on 12 May 2012).

Allan, C. (2007) 'This Unfair Smoking Ban will mean Fuming on the Wards', *Guardian*. Available online at www.theguardian.com/society/2007/feb/07/smoking.socialcare (accessed on 1 April 2015).

Allen, A. (1999) *The Power of Feminist Theory: Domination, resistance, solidarity*, Colorado: Westview Press.

Althusser, L. (2001) *Lenin and Philosophy and Other Essays*, New York: Monthly Review Press.

Amara, P. (2014) 'Smokers and the Obese in Devon will be Barred from Operations as

Part of NHS Cost Cutting', *Independent*, 3 April 2014. Available online at www.independent.co.uk/life-style/health-and-families/health-news/smokers-and-the-obese-in-devon-will-be-barred-from-operations-as-part-of-nhs-cost-cutting-9902044.html.

Anderson, J. (1996) 'Yes, but is it Empowerment? Initiation, implementation and outcomes of community action' in Humphries, B. (ed.) *Critical Perspectives on Empowerment*, Birmingham: Venture Press, pp. 105–127.

Appleby, L. (2007) 'Letter to the Guardian', *Guardian*. Available online at www.theguardian.com/society/2007/feb/14/guardiansocietysupplement (accessed on 1 April 2015).

Arendt, H. (1998 [1958]) *The Human Condition*, Chicago: University of Chicago Press.

Baistow, K. (1995) 'Liberation and Regulation? Some paradoxes of empowerment', *Critical Social Policy*, vol. 14, pp. 34–46.

Baggott, R. (2005) 'From Sickness to Health: Public health in England', *Public, Money and Management*, vol. 25, pp. 229–236.

Bar-On, A. (1999) 'Social Work and the "Missionary Zeal to Whip the Heathen Along the Path of Righteousness"', *British Journal of Social Work*, vol. 29, pp. 5–26.

Bartky, S. (1990) 'Foucault, Femininity and the Modernization of Patriarchal Power' in Bartky, S. *Femininity and Domination*, New York: Routledge, pp. 63–82.

Bauman, Z. (1982) *Memories of Class: The pre-history and after-life of class*, London: Routledge and Kegan Paul.

Bauman, Z. (2013) *Identity*, Cambridge: Polity Press.

Beauchamp, D. (1997) 'Lifestyle, Public Health and Paternalism' in Sidell, M., Jones, L., Katz, J. and Peberdy, A. (eds) *Debates and Dilemmas in Promoting Health: A reader*, Hampshire: Palgrave, pp. 297–305.

Beck, U. (1992) *Risk Society: Towards a new modernity*, London: Sage.

Becker, H. (1963) *Outsiders: Studies in the sociology of deviance*, New York: Free Press.

Behlmer, G. (1982) *Child Abuse and Moral Reform in England 1870–1908*, Stanford: Stanford University Press.

Benzeval, M., Judge, K. and Whitehead, M. (eds) (1995) *Tackling Inequalities in Health: An agenda for action*, London: King's Fund.

Berlin, I. (1969) *Four Essays on Liberty*, Oxford: Oxford University Press.

Beuret, K. and Stoker, G. (1986) 'The Labour Party and Neighbourhood Decentralisation: Flirtation or commitment?' *Critical Social Policy*, October 1986, vol. 6, 17, pp. 4–22.

Bhaskar, R. (1989) *Reclaiming Reality: A Critical introduction to contemporary philosophy*, London: Verso.

Black, D. (1980) *Report of the Working Group on Inequalities in Health*, London: DHSS.

Bland, R.E. (1997) 'Keyworkers Re-examined: Good practice, quality of care and empowerment in residential care of older people', *British Journal of Social Work*, vol. 27, pp. 585–603.

Bolen, R. (2001) *Child Sexual Abuse: Its scope and our failure*, New York: Springer.

Bourdieu, P. (1984) *Distinction: A social critique of the judgement of taste*, Massachusetts: Harvard University Press.

Bourdieu, P. (1990) *In Other Words: Essays towards a reflexive sociology*, Stanford: Stanford University Press.

Boushel, M. (1994) 'The Protective Environment of Children: Towards a framework for anti-oppressive, cross-cultural and cross national understanding', *British Journal of Social Work*, vol. 24, pp. 173–190.

Braye, S. and Preston-Shoot, M. (1990) 'On Teaching and Applying the Law in Social Work: It is not that simple', *British Journal of Social Work*, vol. 20, pp. 333–353.

Brown, K. (2015) *Vulnerability and Young People: Care and social control in policy and practice*, Bristol: The Policy Press.

Browne, J. (1996) 'Unasked Questions or Unheard Answers? Policy development in child sexual abuse', *British Journal of Social Work*, vol. 26, pp. 37–52.

Bunton, R. (1990) 'Regulating Our Favourite Drug' in Abbott, P. and Payne, G. (eds) *New Directions in the Sociology of Health*, London: Falmer, pp. 104–117.

Burrows, R., Nettleton, S. and Bunton, R. (1994) 'Sociology and Health Promotion: Health, risk and consumption under late modernism' in Bunton, R., Nettleton, S. and Burrows, R. (eds) *The Sociology of Health Promotion: Critical analyses of consumption, lifestyle and risk*, London: Routledge, pp. 1–12.

Butler, J. (2006 [1990]) *Gender Trouble*, London: Routledge.

Cabinet Office (2010) *Applying Behavioural Insight to Health*, London: Cabinet Office.

Calder, M. (1995) 'Child Protection: Balancing, paternalism and partnership', *British Journal of Social Work*, vol. 25, pp. 749–766.

Callon, M. and Latour, B. (1981) 'Unscrewing the Big leviathan: How actors macrostructure reality and sociologists help them to do so' in Knorr-Cetina, K.D. and Cicourel, A. (eds) *Advances in Social Theory and Methodology: Towards an integration of micro and macro-sociologies*, London: Routledge and Kegan Paul, pp. 227–303.

Cambridge Dictionary (no date) 'Consciousness Raising'. Available online at http://dictionary. cambridge.org/dictionary/british/consciousness-raising (accessed on 24 May 2015).

Camerer, C., Issacharoff, S., Loewenstein, G., O'Donoghue, T. and Rabin, M. (2003) 'Regulation for Conservatives: Behavioral Economics and the case for "asymmetric paternalism"', *University of Pennsylvania Law Review*, vol. 151, pp. 1211–1254.

Cameron, D. (2009) 'Time to transfer power from the central state to local people', Conservative Party Speeches. Available online at http://conservative-speeches.sayit. mysociety.org/speech/601402 (accessed on 22 May 2010).

Carabine, J. (1996) 'Empowering Sexualities' in Humphries, B. (ed.) *Critical Perspectives on Empowerment*, Birmingham: Venture Press, pp. 17–34.

Carbado, D., Crenshaw, K., Mays, V. and Tomlinson, B. (2013) 'Intersectionality: Mapping the movements of a theory', *Du Bois Review: Social Science Research on Race*, vol. 10, no. 2, pp. 303–312.

Carvel, J. (1987) 'Commons Debate on Health Promotion', *The Lancet*, pp. 1037–1038.

Chandler, D. (2013) 'Freedom vs Necessity in International Relations: Human-centred approaches to security and development', London: Zed Books.

Channel 4 News (2014) 'Heated Row as Anti-Abortion Protesters Confronted Again'. Available online at www.channel4.com/news/abortion-clinic-protests-buffer-zone-london-video (accessed on 11 December 2014).

Cheater, A. (1999) 'Power in the Postmodern Era' in Cheater, A. (ed.) *The Anthropology of Power*, London: Routledge, pp. 1–12.

Cheetham, J. (1979) 'Book Review: *Black Empowerment: Social Work in Oppressed Communities* by Barbara Bryant Solomon, (New York, Columbia University Press, 1976)', *British Journal of Social Work*, vol. 9, pp. 416–417.

Clapton, G., Cree, V. and Smith, M. (2013a) 'Moral Panics and Social Work: Towards a sceptical view of UK child protection', *Critical Social Policy*, vol. 33, no. 2, pp. 197–217.

Clapton, G., Cree, V. and Smith, M. (2013b) 'Moral Panics, Claims-Making and Child Protection in the UK', *British Journal of Social Work*, vol. 43, pp. 803–812.

Clark, C. (1998) 'Self-determination and Paternalism in Community Care: Practice and prospects', *British Journal of Social Work*, vol. 28, pp. 387–402.

Clegg, S.R. (1989) *Frameworks of Power*, London: Sage.

CLG (2008) (Communities and Local Government) 'Communities in Control: Real people, real power', London: HMSO. Available online at www.communities.gov.uk/documents/communities/pdf/886045.pdf (accessed on 24 April 2012).

Cnaan, R.A. (1994) 'The New American Social Work Gospel: Case management of the chronically mentally ill', *British Journal of Social Work*, vol. 24, pp. 533–557.

Cohen, S. (1972) *Folk Devils and Moral Panics*, London: Macgibbon and Kee.

Cohen, S. (2002) *Folk Devils and Moral Panics*, 30th anniversary edition, Oxon: Routledge.

Connolly, M. (1994) 'An Act of Empowerment: The Children Young Persons and their Families Act 1989', *British Journal of Social Work*, vol. 24, pp. 87–100.

Cooper, D. (1967) *Psychiatry and Anti-Psychiatry*, Tavistock, London.

Cooper, J. (1988) 'Book Review', *British Journal of Social Work*, vol. 18, pp. 428–430.

Coote, A. (2010) *Ten Big Questions about the Big Society*, London: New Economics Foundation.

Corby, B., Millar, M. and Young, L. (1996) 'Parental Participation on Child Protection Work: Rethinking the rhetoric', *British Journal of Social Work*, vol. 26, pp. 475–492.

Coulshed, V. (1993) 'Adult Learning: Implications for teaching in social work education', *British Journal of Social Work*, vol. 23, pp. 1–13.

Crenshaw, K. (1989) 'Demarginalizing the Intersection of Race and Sex: A black feminist critique of antidiscrimination doctrine, feminist theory and antiracist politics', *University of Chicago Legal Forum*, vol. 140, pp. 139–167.

Crenshaw, K. (1993) 'Mapping the Margins: Intersectionality, identity politics, and violence against women of color', *Stanford Law Review*, vol. 43, pp. 1241–1299.

Cronin, C. (1996) 'Bourdieu and Foucault on Power and Modernity', *Philosophy and Social Criticism*, vol. 22, pp. 55–85.

Cruikshank, B. (1999) *The Will to Empower: Democratic citizens and other subjects*, New York: Cornell University Press.

Csikszentmihalyi, M. (1990). *Flow: The Psychology of optimal experience*, New York: Harper and Row.

Csikszentmihalyi, M. (1998) *Finding Flow: The psychology of engagement with everyday life*, Basic Books.

CSJ (1994) (Commission on Social Justice) *Social Justice*, London: Vintage.

Cudworth, E. (2015) 'Killing Animals: Sociology, species relations and institutionalized violence' *The Sociological Review*. Available online at http://onlinelibrary.wiley.com/doi/10.1111/1467-954X.12222/abstract;jsessionid=C66855923AEE112E5E62D58D23720A39.f01t01 (accessed on 29 April 2015).

Davison, C., Frankel, S. and Smith, G. (1997) 'The Limits of Lifestyle: Re-assessing "fatalism" in the popular culture of health promotion' in Sidell, M., Jones, L., Katz, J. and Peberdy, A. (eds) *Debates and Dilemmas in Promoting Health: A reader*, Hampshire: Palgrave, pp. 24–32.

de Maria, W. (1992) 'On the Trail of a Radical Pedagogy for Social Work Education', *British Journal of Social Work*, vol. 22, pp. 231–252.

Dean, C.J. (1994) 'The Productive Hypothesis – Foucault, Gender, and the History of Sexuality', *History and Theory*, vol. 33, pp. 271–296.

Dean, M. (1999) *Governmentality: Power and rule in modern society*, London: Sage.

Dermott, T. (2013) 'Direct Action versus Awareness Raising: Why it's not a zero sum game', *Guardian*. Available online at www.theguardian.com/global-development-professionals-network/2013/sep/04/campaigning-to-stop-human-trafficking (accessed on 23 January 2015).

DfT (2011) (Department for Transport) *Behavioural Insights Toolkit*, London: Department for Transport. Available online at www.gov.uk/government/uploads/system/uploads/attachment_data/file/3226/toolkit.pdf (accessed on 18 December 2014).

DHSS (1976a) (Department of Health and Social Security) *Prevention and Health: Everybody's business*, London: HMSO.

DHSS (1976b) (Department of Health and Social Security) *Priorities for Health and Personal Social Services in England*, London: HMSO.

DH/SSI (1991) (Department of Health/Social Services Inspectorate) *Practitioners and Managers' Guide to Care Management and Assessment*, London: HMSO.

DoH (Department of Health) (no date) *Public Health Responsibility Deal*. Available online at https://responsibilitydeal.dh.gov.uk/about/ (accessed on 6 May 2015).

DoH (1976) (Department of Health) *Prevention and Health: Everybody's business*, London: Department of Health.

DoH (1992) (Department of Health) *The Health of the Nation: A strategy for health in England*, London: HMSO.

DoH (1995) (Department of Health, Sub-group of the Chief Medical Officer's Health of the Nation Working Group) *Variations in Health, What Can the NHS Do?* London: Department of Health.

DoH (1997) *The Health of the Nation: A policy assessed* (Executive Summary), London: The Stationery Office. Available online at http://webarchive.nationalarchives.gov.uk/20130107105354/ and www.dh.gov.uk/prod_consum_dh/groups/dh_digitalassets/@dh/@en/documents/digitalasset/dh_4014481.pdf (accessed on 25 February 2015).

DoH (1999) (Department of Health) *Saving Lives: Our healthier nation*, London: Department of Health. Available online at www.gov.uk/government/uploads/system/uploads/attachment_data/file/265576/4386.pdf (accessed on 18 December 2014).

DoH (2004) (Department of Health) *Choosing Health: Making healthy choices easier*, London: Department of Health.

Dolan, P., Hallsworth, M., Halpern, D., King, D and Vlaev, I. (2010) *Mindspace: Influencing behaviour through public policy*, London: Cabinet Office and Institute of Government. Available online at www.instituteforgovernment.org.uk/sites/default/files/publications/MINDSPACE.pdf (accessed on 7 October 2014).

Dominelli, L. (1989) 'Betrayal of Trust: A feminist analysis of power relationships in incest abuse and its relevance for social work practice', *British Journal of Social Work*, vol. 19, pp. 291–307.

Dominelli, L. (1996) 'Deprofessionalizing Social Work: Anti-oppressive practice, competences and postmodernism', *British Journal of Social Work*, vol. 25, pp. 153–175.

Durkheim, E. (1938) *The Rules of Sociological Method*, New York: The Free Press.

Dworkin, G. (2014) 'Paternalism', *Stanford Encyclopaedia of Philosophy*. Available online at http://plato.stanford.edu/entries/paternalism/ (accessed on 8 December 2014).

Ebrahim, S. (1995) 'Public Health Implications of Ageing', *Journal of the Royal College of Physicians of London*, vol. 29, no. 3, pp. 207–215.

Ehrenreich, N. (2002) 'Subordination and Symbiosis: Mechanisms of mutual support between subordinating systems', *UMKC Law Review*, no. 71, pp. 251–324.

Engels, F. (1969 [1845]) *The Conditions of the Working Class in England in 1844*, Moscow: Panther Books.

Engels, F. (2004 [1884]) *The Origins of the Family, Private Property and the State*, New South Wales: Resistance Books.

Fanon, F. (1963) *The Wretched of the Earth*, New York: Grove Press.

Farrell, H. and Shalizi, C. (2011) 'Nudge Polices are Another Name for Coercion', *New*

Scientist, issue 2837. Available online at www.newscientist.com/article/mg21228 376.500-nudge-policies-are-another-name-for-coercion.html (accessed on 3 November 2014).

Fielden, M.A. (1990) 'Reminiscence as a Therapeutic Intervention with Sheltered Housing Residents: A comparative study', *British Journal of Social Work*, vol. 20, pp. 21–44.

Fitzpatrick, M. (2001) 'The Tyranny of Health: Doctors and the regulation of lifestyle', London: Routledge.

Fook, J. (2002) *Social Work: Critical theory and practice*, London: Sage.

Forbes, J. and Sashidharan, P. (1997) 'User Involvement in Services: Incorporation or challenge?' *British Journal of Social Work*, vol. 27, pp. 481–498.

Forgacs, D. (ed.) (1999) *The Antonio Gramsci Reader: Selected writings 1916–1935*, London: Lawrence and Wishart.

Foucault, M. (1980) *Power/Knowledge: Selected interviews and other writings 1972–1977*, Essex: Pearson Education.

Foucault, M. (1982) 'The Subject and Power', *Critical Inquiry*, vol. 8, pp. 777–795.

Foucault, M. (1983) 'The Subject and Power' in Dreyfus, H.L. and Rabinow, P. (eds) *Michel Foucault: Beyond structuralism and hermeneutics*, Chicago: University of Chicago Press, pp. 208–226.

Foucault, M. (1990) *The History of Sexuality*, vol. 1, London: Penguin.

Foucault, M. (1991a [1977]) *Discipline and Punish: The birth of the prison*, London: Penguin.

Foucault, M. (1991b) *Remarks on Marx: Conversations with Duccio Trombadori*, New York: Semiotexte.

Foucault, M. (1991c) 'Nietzsche, Genealogy, History' in Rabinow, P. (ed.) *The Foucault Reader: An introduction to Foucault's thought*, London: Penguin.

Fraser, N. and Gordon, L. (1994) 'A Genealogy of Dependency: Tracing a keyword of the US welfare system', *Signs*, vol. 19, pp. 309–336.

Friere, P. (1970) *The Pedagogy of the Oppressed*, New York: Continuum.

Furedi, F. (2013a) *Moral Crusades in an Age of Mistrust: The Jimmy Savile scandal*, Hampshire: Palgrave-Macmillan.

Furedi, F. (2013b) 'The Moral Lynching of Barbara Hewson', *Spiked*. Available online at www.spiked-online.com/site/article/13612/ (accessed on 15 May 2013).

Furedi, F. (2013c) 'I Don't Want to Have my Awareness Raised, Thanks', *Spiked*. Available online at www.spiked-online.com/newsite/article/i_dont_want_to_have_my_ awareness_raised_thanks/13770#.VMHZy2BybRM (accessed on 14 January 2015).

Giddens, A. (1994) *Beyond Left and Right: The future of radical politics*, Oxford: The Polity Press.

Giddens, A. (2000) *The Third Way and its Critics*, Cambridge: Polity Press.

Gilbert, N. (1997) 'Advocacy Research and Social Policy', *Crime and Justice*, vol. 22, pp. 101–148.

Goddard, E. and Green, H. (2005) *Smoking and Drinking among Adults, 2004*, General Household Survey 2004, London: ONS.

Gomm, R. (1993) 'Issues of Power in Social Welfare' in Walmsley, J., Reynolds, J., Shakespeare, P. and Woolfe, R. (eds) *Health, Welfare and Practice: Reflecting on roles and relationships*, London: Sage, pp. 131–138.

Goodwin, T. (2012) 'Why We Should Reject "Nudge"', *Politics*, vol. 32, pp. 85–92.

Gorski, P.C. and Goodman, R.D. (2011) 'Is There a "Hierarchy of Oppression" in U.S. Multicultural Teacher Education Coursework?' *Action in Teacher Education*, vol. 33, pp. 455–475.

Graham, M.J. (1999) 'The African-Centred Worldview: Developing a paradigm for social work', *British Journal of Social Work*, vol. 29, pp. 251–267.

Gramsci, A. (1971) *Selections from Prison Notebook*, London: Lawrence and Wishart.

Groce, N.E. (1993) 'A Community's Adaptation to Deafness' in Walmsley, J., Reynolds, J., Shakespeare, P. and Woolfe, R. (eds) *Health, Welfare and Practice: Reflecting on roles and relationships*, London: Sage, pp. 144–146.

Guidroz, K and Berger, M. (2009) 'A Conversation with Founding Scholars of Intersectionality: Kimberlie Crenshaw, Nira Yuval-Davis, and Michelle Fine' in Berger, M. and Guidroz, K. (eds) *The Intersectional Approach: Transforming the academy through race, class and gender*, Carolina; University of North Carolina Press, pp. 61–78.

Gutfield, G. (2011) 'Raise Awareness of Raising Awareness of Raising Awareness', *Huffington Post*. Available online at www.huffingtonpost.com/greg-gutfeld/raise-awareness-of-raisin_b_7573.html (accessed on 12 January 2015).

Haaken, J. (2000) *Pillar of Salt: Gender, memory and the perils of looking back*, New Jersey: Rutgers University Press.

Habermas, J. (1984) *The Theory of Communicative Action (Vol. 1): Reason and the rationalisation of society*, London: Heinemann.

Habermas, J. (1987) *The Philosophical Discourse of Modernity: Twelve Lectures*, Cambridge, MA: MIT Press.

Hall, S., Critcher, C., Jefferson, T., Clarke, J. and Roberts, B. (1978) *Policing the Crisis: Mugging, the state and law and order*, London: Macmillan.

Halpern, D., Bates, C., Mulgan, G., Aldridge, S., Beales, G. and Heathfield, A. (2004) *Personal Responsibility and Changing Behaviour: The state of knowledge and its implications for public policy*, London: Cabinet Office, Prime Minister's Strategy Unit. Available online at http://webarchive.nationalarchives.gov.uk/+/http:/ and www.cabinetoffice.gov.uk/media/cabinetoffice/strategy/assets/pr2.pdf (accessed on 6 April 2015).

Harker, L., Jutte, S., Murphy, T., Bentley, H., Miller, P. and Fitch, K. (2012) *How Safe Are Our Children*, London: NSPCC. Available online at www.nspcc.org.uk/Inform/research/findings/howsafe/how-safe-2013-report_wdf95435.pdf (accessed on 13 June 2012).

Hartsock, N.C.M. (1998) *The Feminist Standpoint Revisited and Other Essays*, Oxford: Westview Press.

Hastings, R. (2014) 'Nappies Could Contain Messages to get Parents Talking to Babies', *Independent*, 23 September 2014.

Hatfield, B., Huxley, P. and Mohamad, H. (1992) 'Accommodation and Employment: A survey into the circumstances and expressed needs of users of mental health services in a Northern town', *British Journal of Social Work*, vol. 22, pp. 61–73.

Hayek, F.A. (1960) *The Constitution of Liberty*, London: Routledge.

Heartfield, J. (2002) *The 'Death of the Subject' Explained*, Sheffield: Sheffield Hallam University Press.

Heath, I. (1995) *The Mystery of General Practice*, London: Nuffield Provincial Hospitals Trust. Available online at www.nuffieldtrust.org.uk/sites/files/nuffield/publication/The_Mystery_of_General_Practice.pdf (accessed on 16 March 2015).

Hewson, B. (2013) 'Yewtree is Destroying the Rule of Law', *Spiked*. Available online at www.spiked-online.com/site/article/13604/ (accessed on 11 May 2013).

Hill Collins, P. (1990) *Black Feminist Thought: Knowledge, consciousness and the politics of empowerment*, London; Hyman.

Hobbes, T. (2008 [1651]) *Leviathan*, Oxford: Oxford University Press.

Honneth, A. (1991) *The Critique of Power: Reflective stages in critical social theory*, London: MIT Press.

hooks, b. (1981). *Ain't I a Woman? Black Women and Feminism*, Boston, MA: South End Press.

hooks, b. (2015) *Feminist Theory: From margin to center*, 3rd edition, Abingdon: Routledge.

Howe, D. (1994) 'Modernity, Postmodernity and Social Work', *British Journal of Social Work*, vol. 24, pp. 513–532.

Hudson, A. (1989) 'Changing Perspectives: Feminism, gender and social work' in Langan, M. and Lee, P. (eds) *Radical Social Work Today*, London: Unwin Hyman, pp. 70–96.

Hughes, B. (1993) 'A Model for the Comprehensive Assessment of Older people and their Carers', *British Journal of Social Work*, vol. 23, pp. 345–364.

Hugman, R. (1991) 'Organization and Professionalism: The social work agenda in the 1990s', *British Journal of Social Work*, vol. 21, pp. 199–216.

Hume, M. (2015) *Trigger Warning: Is fear of being offensive killing free speech*, London: William Collins.

Humphries, B. (1996) 'Contradictions in the Culture of Empowerment' in Humphries, B. (ed.) *Critical Perspectives on Empowerment*, Birmingham: Venture Press, pp. 1–16.

Humphries, B. (1997) 'Reading Social Work: Competing discourses in the rules and requirements for the diploma in social work', *British Journal of Social Work*, vol. 27, pp. 641–658.

Humphries, B. (2004) 'An Unacceptable Role for Social Work: Implementing immigration policy', *British Journal of Social Work*, vol. 34, pp. 93–107.

Hunter, D. (2007) 'Public Health: Historical context and current agenda' in Scriven, A. and Garman, S. *Public Health: Social context and action*, Maidenhead: Open University Press, pp. 8–19.

Hunter, D., Fulop, N. and Warner, M. (2000) *From 'Health of the Nation' to 'Our Healthier Nation'*, European Centre for Health Policy, Policy Learning Curve Series, no. 2. Available online at www.euro.who.int/__data/assets/pdf_file/0007/119932/E70042.pdf (accessed on 25 February 2015).

Ingram, D. (1994) 'Foucault and Habermas on the Subject of Reason' in Gutting, G. (ed.) *The Cambridge Companion to Foucault*, Cambridge: Cambridge University Press, pp. 215–261.

Isin, E.F. (2004) 'The Neurotic Citizen', *Citizenship Studies*, vol. 8, pp. 217–235.

Jackson, S. (1996) 'Obituary of Baroness Faithful 1910–1996', *British Journal of Social Work*, vol. 26, pp. 447–450.

James, W. (1999) 'Empowering Ambiguities' in Cheater, A. (ed.) *The Anthropology of Power*, London: Routledge, pp. 13–27.

Jankowski, K.A. (1997) *Deaf Empowerment: Emergence, struggle and rhetoric*, Washington: Gallaudet University Press.

Jenkins, P. (1992) *Intimate Enemies: Moral panics in contemporary Great Britain*, New York: Aldine de Gruyter.

Jochelson, K. (2006) 'Smoke-Free Legislation and Mental Health Units: The challenges ahead', *British Journal of Psychiatry*, no. 188, pp. 479–480.

John, P., Cotterill, S., Moseley, A., Richardson, L., Smith, G., Stoker, G. and Wales, C. (2013) *Nudge, Nudge, Think, Think: Experimenting with ways to change civic behaviour*, London: Bloomsbury.

Jones, R., Pykett, J. and Whitehead, M. (2011) 'Governing Temptation: Changing behaviour in an age of libertarian paternalism', *Progress in Human Geography*, vol. 35, pp. 483–501.

Jones, R., Pykett, J. and Whitehead, M. (2013) *Changing Behaviours: On the rise of the psychological state*, Cheltenham: Edward Elgar publishing.

Jupp, B., Briscoe, I., Wade, J., Perri 6, Stanley, R. and Bentley, T. (1995) *Missionary Government*, London: Demos.

Kelly, M. and Charlton, B. (1994) 'The Modern and the Postmodern in Health Promotion' in Bunton, R., Nettleton, S. and Burrows, R. (eds) *The Sociology of Health Promotion: Critical analyses of consumption, lifestyle and risk*, London: Routledge, pp. 1–12.

Kendall, S. (1998) *Health and Empowerment: Research and practice*, London: Arnold.

King, M. (2007) 'Mass Media, Lifestyle and Public Health' in Scriven, A. and Garman, S. *Public Health: Social context and action*, Maidenhead, Open University Press, pp. 95–104.

Ladd, P. (2003) *Understanding Deaf Culture: In search of Deafhood*, Bristol: Multilingual Matters.

Lakoff, G. and Johnson, G. (2003) *Metaphors We Live By*, Chicago: University of Chicago Press.

Lalonde, M. (1974) *A New Perspective on the Health of Canadians*, Ottawa: Ministry of Supplies and Services.

Langan, M. (1998) 'The Legacy of Radical Social Work' in Adams, R., Dominelli, L. and Payne, M. (eds) *Social Work: Themes, Issues and Critical Debates*, London: Palgrave, pp. 209–217.

Leadbetter, M. (2002) 'Empowerment and Advocacy' in Adams, R., Dominelli, L. and Payne, M. (eds) *Social Work: Themes, Issues and Critical Debates,* 2nd edition, Hampshire: Palgrave, pp. 200–208.

Lenin, V.I. (1994 [1917]) *The State and Revolution*, London: Junius.

Lewis, J., Bernstock, P., Bovell, V. and Wookey, F. (1997) 'Implementing Care Management: Issues in relation to the new community care', *British Journal of Social Work*, vol. 27, pp. 5–24.

Lloyd, M. (2001) 'The Politics of Disability and Feminism: Discord or synthesis', *Sociology*, vol. 35, no. 3, pp. 715–728.

Lorde, A. (1983) 'There is No Hierarchy of Oppression', *Bulletin: Homophobia and Education*, vol. 14, p. 9.

Lucas, J. (2006) 'Book Review', *British Journal of Social Work*, vol. 36, pp. 689–691.

Lukes, S. (2005 [1974]) *Power: A radical view*, 2nd edition, Basingstoke: Palgrave.

Lupton, C. (1998) 'User Empowerment or Family Self-Reliance? The Family Group Conference Model', *British Journal of Social Work*, vol. 28, pp. 107–128.

Lutz, H. (2002) 'Intersectional Analysis: A way out of multiple dilemmas', paper presented at the International Sociological Association conference, Brisbane, Australia.

Machiavelli, N. (2009 [1532]) *The Prince*, Toronto: Prohyptikon Publishing.

Malik, A. (2014) 'DWP Orders Man to Work Without Pay for Company that Let Him go', *Guardian.* Available online at www.theguardian.com/society/2014/nov/03/dwp-benefits-electrician-work-placement-labour (accessed on 7 November 2014).

Marcuse, H. (2008) *A Study on Authority*, London: Verso (first published 1936).

Marx, K. and Engels, F. (1970 [1846]) *The German Ideology*, London: Lawrence and Wishart.

Marx, K. and Engels, F. (1996 [1872]) *The Communist Manifesto*, London: Junius.

Mather, S. and Mitchell, R. (1994) 'Communication Abuse: A sociolinguistic perspective' in Snider, B. (ed.) *Post Milan ASL and English Literacy: Issues, trends and research*, Washington: Gallaudet University, pp. 89–117.

McCabe, A. (2010) 'Below the Radar in a Big Society? Reflections on community engagement, empowerment and social action in a changing policy context', *Third Sector Research Centre*, Working Paper 51.

McCall, L. (2009) 'The Complexity of Intersectionality' in Grabham, E., Cooper, D., Krishnadas, J. and Herman, D. (eds) *Intersectionality and Beyond: Law, power and the politics of location*, Abingdon: Routledge, pp. 49–76.

McKeown, R. (2014) 'Petition is launched to save Burger King in Southampton General Hospital from closing', *Southern Daily Echo*. Available online at www.dailyecho.co.uk/news/11620844.Fight_launched_to_save_Burger_King_at_hospital/ (accessed on 12 December 2014).

McLaughlin, J. (2003) *Feminist Social and Political Theory: Contemporary debates and dialogues*, Hampshire: Palgrave Macmillan, pp. 91–103.

McLaughlin, K. (2008) *Social Work, Politics and Society: From radicalism to orthodoxy*, Bristol: The Polity Press.

McLaughlin, K. (2012) *Surviving Identity: Vulnerability and the psychology of recognition*, London: Routledge.

McLaughlin, K. (2015) 'Politics as Social Work: The micromanagement of behaviour in the new millennium' in Palattiyil, G., Sidhva, D. and Chakrabarti, M. (eds) *Social Work in a Global Context: Issues and Challenges*, London: Routledge.

McNay, L. (1994) *Foucault: A critical introduction*, Cambridge: Polity Press.

McSmith, A. (2010) 'First Obama, Now Cameron Embraces Nudge Theory', *Independent*. Available online at www.independent.co.uk/news/uk/politics/first-obama-now-cameron-embraces-nudge-theory-2050127.html (accessed on 16 December 2014).

Mill, J.S. (2008 [1859]) *On Liberty and Other Essays*, Oxford: Oxford University Press.

Moore, S. (2010) *Ribbon Culture: Charity, compassion and public awareness*, London: Palgrave.

Morgan, A. and Popay, J. (2007) 'Community Participation for Health; Reducing health inequalities and building social capital' in Scriven, A. and Garman, S. *Public Health: Social context and action*, Maidenhead, Open University Press, pp. 154–165.

Morris, J. (1991) *Pride against Prejudice: Transforming attitudes to disability*, London: The Women's Press.

Morrison, K. (2006) *Marx, Durkheim, Weber: Formations of modern social thought*, 2nd edition, London: Sage.

Murphy, P. (2014) 'Are You Prepared to Join the Hairy Legs Movement?', *Independent*. Available online at www.independent.ie/life/are-you-prepared-to-join-the-hairy-legs-movement-30433200.html (accessed on 22 April 2015).

Naik, D. (1993) 'Towards an Anti-Racist Curriculum in Social Work Training' in Walmsley, J., Reynolds, J., Shakespeare, P. and Woolfe, R. (eds) *Health, Welfare and Practice: Reflecting on roles and relationships*, London: Sage, pp. 83–89.

Nettleton, S. and Bunton, R. (1994) 'Sociological Critiques of Health Promotion' in Bunton, R., Nettleton, S. and Burrows, R. (eds) *The Sociology of Health Promotion: Critical analyses of consumption, lifestyle and risk*, London: Routledge, pp. 41–59.

Nigan, A. (1996) 'Marxism and Power', *Social Scientist*, vol. 24, pp. 3–22.

NSPCC (2011) *Reports and Accounts 2010/11*, NSPCC. Available online at www.nspcc.org.uk/what-we-do/about-the-nspcc/annual-report/annual-report-archive/annual-review-2010_wdf84903.pdf (accessed on 9 October 2011).

NSPCC (2012a) 'Nearly a Thousand Registered Child Sex Abusers Reoffended', NSPCC press release. Available online at www.nspcc.org.uk/news-and-views/media-centre/

press-releases/2012/12-11-18-child-sex-abusers-reoffend/registered-child-abusers-reoffend_wdn92904.html (accessed on 15 December 2012).

NSPCC (2012b) 'Savile Case Prompts Surge in Calls to NSPCC about Children Suffering Sexual Abuse Right Now', NSPCC press release. Available online at www.nspcc.org.uk/news-and-views/media-centre/press-releases/2012/12-10-savile-case-prompts-surge-in-calls/savile-case-prompts-surge-in-calls-to-nspcc_wdn92545.html (accessed on 15 December 2012).

NSPCC (2012c) 'NSPCC: Babies still at high risk five years after the death of Baby Peter', NSPCC press release. Available online at www.nspcc.org.uk/news-and-views/media-centre/press-releases/2012/12-08-01-babies-still-at-high-risk/babies-still-at-high-risk_wdn91131.html (accessed on 15 December 2012).

NSPCC (2012d) 'NSPCC Warns of Child Neglect Crisis as Reports to its Helpline Double', NSPCC press release. Available online at www.nspcc.org.uk/news-and-views/media-centre/press-releases/2012/12-06-11-neglect-theme-launch/child-neglect-crisis_wdn89914.html (accessed on 15 December 2012).

NSPCC (2012e) 'Children Who Witness Family Violence More Likely to Carry a Weapon, Seriously Harm Someone or be Excluded from School', NSPCC press release. Available online at www.nspcc.org.uk/news-and-views/media-centre/press-releases/2012/12-05-31-children-witnessing-family-violence/children-witnessing-family-violence_wdn89979.html (accessed on 15 December 2012).

NSPCC (2012f) '"Sexting" from Peers More Concerning than "Stranger Danger" to Young People warns the NSPCC', NSPCC press release. Available online at www.nspcc.org.uk/news-and-views/media-centre/press-releases/2012/12-05-16-sexting-from-peers/sexting-from-peers_wdn89458.html (accessed on 15 December 2012).

NSPCC (2012g) 'New Mums Struggling to Cope Warns NSPCC', NSPCC press release. Available online at www.nspcc.org.uk/news-and-views/media-centre/press-releases/2012/12-05-11-new-mums-struggling/new-mums-struggling_wdn89327.html (accessed on 15 December 2012).

NSPCC (2012h) 'Caught in a Trap: The impact of grooming in 2012'. Available online at www.nspcc.org.uk/news-and-views/our-news/nspcc-news/12-11-12-grooming-report/caught-in-a-trap-pdf_wdf92793.pdf (accessed on 15 May 2013).

NSPCC (2012i) *Annual Report 2011/12.* Available online at www.nspcc.org.uk/what-we-do/about-the-nspcc/annual-report/annual-report-2012/annual-report-2012-pdf_wdf92210.pdf (accessed on 6 August 2012).

NSPCC (2013) 'NSPCC Warns of E-Safety "Timebomb"', NSPCC press release. Available online at www.nspcc.org.uk/news-and-views/media-centre/press-releases/2013/13-02-05-NSPCC-warns-of-esafety-timebomb/NSPCC-warns-of-esafety-timebomb_wdn94135.html (accessed on 12 April 2013).

Oakely, A. (1989) 'Smoking in Pregnancy: Smoke screen or risk factor? Towards a materialistic analysis', *Sociology of Health and Illness*, vol. 11, pp. 311–355.

Oliver, M. (1996) *Understanding Disability: From theory to practice*, Basingstoke: Palgrave.

Oxford English Dictionary (1983) *The Shorter Oxford English Dictionary*, vol. 1, London: Guild Publishing.

Parish, R. (1994) 'Health Promotion: Rhetoric and reality' in Bunton, R., Nettleton, S. and Burrows, R. (eds) *The Sociology of Health Promotion: Critical analyses of consumption, lifestyle and risk*, London: Routledge, pp. 13–23.

Parsloe, P. (1996a) 'Introduction' in Parsloe, P. (ed.) *Pathways to Empowerment*, Birmingham: Venture Press, pp. xvii–xxii.

Parsloe, P. (1996b) 'Empowerment in Social Work Practice' in Parsloe, P. (ed.) *Pathways to Empowerment*, Birmingham: Venture Press, pp. 1–10.

Parsons, T. (1957) 'The Distribution of Power in American Society', *World Politics*, vol. 10, pp. 123–143.

Parsons, T. (1963) 'On the Concept of Power', *Proceedings of the American Philosophical Society*, vol. 107, no. 3, pp. 232–262.

Peterson, A. and Lupton, D. (1996) *The New Public Health*, London: Sage.

Powell, F. (2013) *The Politics of Civil Society*, 2nd edition, Bristol: The Policy Press.

Prasad, R. (2003) 'Sound and Fury', *Guardian*. Available online at www.theguardian.com/society/2003/mar/19/guardiansocietysupplement5 (accessed on 29 April 2015).

Pritchard, C. and Williams, R. (2010) 'Comparing Possible "Child-Abuse-Related-Deaths" in England and Wales with the Major Developed Countries 1974–2006: Signs of progress?', *British Journal of Social Work*, vol. 40, pp. 1700–1718.

Rabinow, P. (1991) (ed.) *The Foucault Reader: An introduction to Foucault's thought*, London: Penguin.

Radford, L., Corral, S., Bradley, C., Fisher, H., Bassett, C., Howatt, N. and Collishaw, S. (2011) *Child Abuse and Neglect in the UK Today*, London: NSPCC. Available online at www.nspcc.org.uk/Inform/research/findings/child_abuse_neglect_research_PDF_wdf84181.pdf (accessed on 2 February 2012).

Ramazanoglu, C. and Holland, J. (1993) 'Women's Sexuality and Men's Appropriation of Desire', in Ramazanoglu, C. (ed.) *Up Against Foucault: Explorations of some tensions between Foucault and feminism*, London: Routledge, pp. 239–264.

Ramon, S. (1995) 'Slovenian Social Work: A case study of unexpected developments in the post 1990 period', *British Journal of Social Work*, vol. 25, pp. 513–528.

Rawls, J. (1971) *A Theory of Justice*, Massachusetts: Harvard University Press.

Rayner, J. (1999) 'Why this NSPCC Advert is Harmful to Children', *Observer*. Available online at www.theguardian.com/Archive/Article/0,4273,3890641,00..html (accessed on 24 April 2014).

Rogowski, J. (2010) *Social Work: The Rise and fall of a profession*, Bristol: The Policy Press.

Rollins, J. (1985) *Between Women: Domestics and their employers*, Philadelphia: Temple University Press.

Rose, N. (1990) *Governing the Soul: The shaping of the private self*, London: Routledge.

Rose, N. (1996) 'Psychiatry as a political science: Advanced liberalism and the administration of risk', *History of the Human Sciences*, vol. 9, no. 2, pp. 1–23.

Rosen, R. (2000) *The World Split Open: How the modern women's movement changed America*, New York: Viking.

Rossetti, F. (1987) 'Book Review' *British Journal of Social Work*, vol. 17, pp. 329–331.

Rousseau, J.J. (1998 [1792]) *The Social Contract*, Hertfordshire: Wordsworth.

Ryan, P.J. (1986) 'The Contribution of Formal and Informal Systems of Intervention to the Alleviation of Depression in Young Mothers', *British Journal of Social Work*, vol. 16, pp. 71–82.

Sarachild, K. (1970). 'A Program for Feminist "Consciousness Raising"', *Notes From the Second Year: Women's Liberation: Major Writings of the Radical Feminists*, pp. 78–80.

Sawicki, J. (1991) *Disciplining Foucault: Feminism, Power and the Body*, London: Routledge.

Sayce, L. (2000) *From Psychiatric Patient to Citizen: Overcoming discrimination and social exclusion*, Basingstoke: Palgrave.

Secrett, C. and Bullock, S. (2002) 'Sustainable Development and Health' in Adams, L.,

Amos, M. and Munro, J. (eds) *Promoting Health: Politics and Practice*, London: Sage. pp. 34–45.

Seedhouse, D. (1997) *Health promotion: Philosophy, prejudice and practice*, Chichester: Wiley.

Seligman, M. (2002) *Authentic Happiness: Using the new positive psychology to realize your potential for lasting fulfilment*, New York: Free Press.

Seligman, M. and Csikszentmihalyi, M. (2000) 'Positive Psychology: An introduction', *American Psychologist*, vol. 55, pp. 5–14.

Sen, A. (2009) *The Idea of Justice*, Massachusetts: Harvard: University Press.

Service, P. (1985) 'Book Review', *British Journal of Social Work*, vol. 15, pp. 433–434.

Seymour, B. and Vlaev, I. (2012) 'Can, and Should, Behavioural Neuroscience Influence Public Policy?' *Trends in Cognitive Sciences*, vol. 12, no. 9, pp. 449–451.

Simon, H. (1957) *Models of Man: Social and rational*, London: John Wiley and Sons.

Skinner, Q. (1978a) *The Foundations of Modern Political Thought, The Renaissance*, Cambridge: Cambridge University Press.

Skinner, Q. (1978b) *The Foundations of Modern Political Thought, The Age of Reformation*, Cambridge: Cambridge University Press.

Smith, H. and Brown, H. (1992) 'Defending Community Care: Can normalization do the job?' *British Journal of Social Work*, vol. 22, pp. 685–693.

Smith, L. (2015) 'Everyday Sexism's Laura Bates: "Awareness-raising has become a worldwide movement for equality"', *Guardian*. Available online at www.ibtimes.co.uk/everyday-sexisms-laura-bates-awareness-raising-has-become-worldwide-movement-equality-1496498 (accessed on 25 May 2015).

Smith, R. (2010) 'Social Work, Risk, Power', *Sociological Research online*, vol. 15, Available online at www.socresonline.org.uk/15/1/4.html (accessed on 13 November 2013).

Solomon, A. (1994) 'Deaf is Beautiful', *New York Times Magazine*, 28 August 1994.

Solomon, B.B. (1976) *Black Empowerment: Social work in oppressed communities*, New York: Columbia University Press.

Sowards, K. and Renegar, V. (2004) 'The Rhetorical Functions Of Consciousness-Raising in Third Wave Feminism', *Communication Studies*, vol. 55, no. 4 (Winter 2004), pp. 535–552. Available online at http://digitalcommons.utep.edu/cgi/viewcontent.cgi?article=1003&context=stacey_sowards (accessed on 24 May 2015).

Spivak, G. (1987) *In Other Worlds: Essays in cultural politics*, New York: Taylor and Francis.

Spivak, G. (1996) *The Spivak Reader: Selected works of Gayati Chakravorty Spivak,* Landry, D. and Maclean, G. (eds) London: Routledge.

Stanford Encyclopedia of Philosophy (no date) 'Paternalism'. Available online at http://plato.stanford.edu/entries/paternalism/ (accessed on 4 December 2014).

Steinmetz, G. (1994) *Regulating the Social: The welfare state and local politics in Imperial Germany*, Princeton: Princeton University Press.

Stevenson, H. and Burke, M. (1991) 'Bureaucratic Logic in New Social Movement Clothing: The limits of health promotion research', *Health Promotion International*, vol. 6, pp. 281–290.

Swingewood, A. (2000) *A Short History of Sociological Thought*, 3rd edition, Hampshire: Palgrave.

Tallis, R. (2011) *Aping Mankind: Neuromania, Darwinitis and the misrepresentation of humanity*, Durham: Acumen.

Taylor, I. (1993) 'Social Work Education', *British Journal of Social Work*, vol. 23, pp. 667–675.

Taylor, M. (2009) 'Left Brain/Right Brain', *Prospect*. Available online at www.prospect-magazine.co.uk/features/left-brain-right-brain (accessed on 4 April 2013).

Thaler, R. and Sunstein, C. (2008) *Nudge: Improving decisions about health*, London: Penguin.

Thomas, M. and Pierson, J. (1995) *Dictionary of Social Work*, London: Collins Educational.

Thompson, N. (2007) *Power and Empowerment*, Lyme Regis: Russell House.

Tiger Beatdown (no date) 'My Feminism will be Intersectional or it will be Bullshit'. Available online at http://tigerbeatdown.com/2011/10/10/my-feminism-will-be-intersectional-or-it-will-be-bullshit/ (accessed on 4 December 2014).

Tones, K. (1997) 'Health Education as Empowerment' in Sidell, M., Jones, L., Katz, J. and Peberdy, A. (eds) *Debates and Dilemmas in Promoting Health: A reader*, Hampshire: Palgrave, pp. 33–42.

Townsend-Bell, E. (2014) 'Ambivalent Intersectionality', *Politics and Gender*, vol. 10, no. 1, pp. 137–142.

Vidal, A. (2014) 'Intersectional Feminism. What the Hell is it? (And Why you Should Care)' *Telegraph*. Available online at www.telegraph.co.uk/women/womens-life/10572435/Intersectional-feminism.-What-the-hell-is-it-And-why-you-should-care.html (accessed on 22 January 2015).

Wai Man, K. (1996) 'Empowerment Practice in Social Work: The case of Hong Kong' in Parsloe, P. *Pathways to Empowerment*, Birmingham: Venture Press, pp. 41–64.

Wainwright, D. (1996) 'The Political Transformation of the Health Inequalities Debate', *Critical Social Policy*, vol. 49, pp. 67–82.

Wang, C. (1992) 'Culture, Meaning and Disability: Injury prevention campaigns and the production of stigma', *Social Science and Medicine*, vol. 35, pp. 1093–1102.

Wanless, D. (2002) *Securing Our Future Health: Taking a long-term view*, London: HM Treasury.

Ward, D. and Mullender, A. (1993) 'Empowerment and Oppression: An indissoluble pairing for contemporary social work' in Walmsley, J., Reynolds, J., Shakespeare, P. and Woolfe, R. (eds) *Health, Welfare and Practice: Reflecting on roles and relationships*, London: Sage, pp. 147–154.

Weber, M. (1978 [1922]) *Economy and Society*, vols 1 and 2, New York: Oxford University Press.

West, P. (2004) *Conspicuous Compassion*, London: Civitas.

Whitehead, M. (1987) *The Health Divide: Inequalities in Health in the 1980s*, London: Health Education Council.

WHO (1948) (World Health Organisation) *WHO Definition of Health*. Available online at www.who.int/about/ definition/en/print.html (accessed on 4 June 2014).

WHO (1984) (World Health Organisation) *Health For All by the Year 2000*, WHO.

WHO (1986) (World Health Organisation) *The Ottawa Charter for Health Promotion*. Available online at www.who.int/healthpromotion/conferences/previous/ottawa/en/ (accessed on 4 June 2014).

WHO (1991) (World Health Organisation) *Targets For Health For All: The health policy for Europe*, WHO.

Wing, D.W. (2010) *Microaggressions in Everyday Life: Race, gender, and sexual orientation*, Hoboken: John Wiley & Sons.

Winnicott, D. (1965) *The Family and Individual Development*, London: Tavistock.

Wolin, S. (1960) *Politics and Vision*, Boston: Little, Brown.

Wright, S. (ed.) (1994) *Anthropology of Organisations*, London: Routledge.

Wrong, D. (1979) *Power: Its forms, bases and uses*, Oxford: Blackwell.

Yeung, K. (2012) 'Nudge as Fudge', *Modern Law Review*, vol. 75, pp. 122–148.

Yon, D. (1999) 'The Discursive Space of Schooling' in Cheater, A. (ed.) *The Anthropology of Power*, London: Routledge, pp. 28–41.

Zamora, D. (2014) 'Can We Criticize Foucault', *Jacobin*. Available online at www.jacobinmag.com/2014/12/foucault-interview/ (accessed on 16 December 2014).

Žižek, S. (2014) 'How WikiLeaks Opened our Eyes to the Illusion of Freedom', *Guardian*. Available online at www.theguardian.com/commentisfree/2014/jun/19/hypocrisy-freedom-julian-assange-wikileaks/print (accessed on 24 June 2014).

Zoido-Oses, P. (2014) 'The Problem with Nudge Policies is that they threaten our Freedom to Choose and Act Well'. Available online at http://blogs.lse.ac.uk/politicsandpolicy/the-problem-with-nudge-policies-freedom-to-choose/ (accessed on 4 May 2015).

Index

Please note that page numbers relating to Notes will be denoted by the letter 'n' and note number following the note.

For Product Safety Concerns and Information please contact our EU
representative GPSR@taylorandfrancis.com
Taylor & Francis Verlag GmbH, Kaufingerstraße 24, 80331 München, Germany